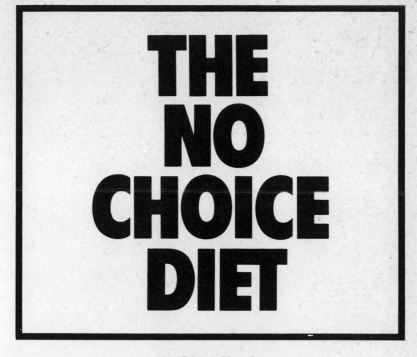

THE NO CHOICE DIET

by **Diane Harris**
Foreword by John Prutting, M.D.

A Tree Communications Edition

Dolphin Books/Doubleday & Company, Inc.
Garden City, New York
1979

Printed in U.S.A.

ISBN 0-385-14517-9

Library of Congress Catalog Card Number 78-067085

Created and produced by Tree Communications, Inc., 250 Park Avenue South, New York, NY

Edited by Maggie Oster, with assistance from Ruth Michel and Mary Clarke/Designed by Sonja Douglas/Exercises performed by Laura P. Hoefler and photographed by David Arky/ Art production by Colette Bellier.

Warning: Check with your physician before starting any exercise program or diet regime. If you have been inactive for a long time, smoke, or are significantly overweight you may need a medical examination, and the physician may want to modify the program.

Why this diet will work

No diet, no matter how good, will work if you can't stick with it. And for most people, sticking with a diet after the first few enthusiastic days gets harder and harder. What the weak-willed among us need is a guiding hand that stays with us all day long, day after day. And that is exactly what the next 208 pages will provide.

Each day for 33 days, you will be given a diet and fitness program that you must follow exactly—morning, daytime, and evening. In addition to three satisfying and nutritionally balanced meals, the plan offers simple exercises to increase your vitality and tone your muscles, beauty hints to polish your looks, and relaxation techniques to reduce tension and combat the temptation to backslide.

Do everything exactly as presented; you will not only lose weight, you will feel more alive and look more attractive day by day. By the time you reach the last page, you will have come to know the guidelines for healthy living; you will have learned to control your eating habits in a way that should help you maintain a proper weight balance.

It is important that you begin this diet on a Monday and make your basic preparations for it on the preceding Saturday. Don't skip ahead in the book. Read each page as you come to it and follow its instructions. When you have completed a page, tear it out and throw it away.

Ready?

Now, tear out this page and throw it away.

A Foreword From A Physician

Let's face it. Obesity is no joke. It's a disease, a common and serious disease from which too many suffer. At one time we used to laugh about jolly fat people. Today, we know that the overweight are vulnerable to numerous ills which can predictably shorten their lives.

It is never easy to lose weight. Genuine motivation must be sustained, and a determined course of self-discipline followed. Despite the many books offered on this subject, often based more on gimmicks than sound nutritional principles, most people just don't stick with a diet. They start out full of resolve and then weaken before reaching their goal. I am confronted with this frequently among my patients. One of the things I like about this book is that it takes a no-nonsense approach. It promises no magical shortcuts. It doesn't pretend that successful dieting can be easy.

What it *does* do is prescribe a 33-day regimen of reduced caloric intake, offering—at the same time—important suggestions for maintaining your psychological determination to slim down. It *commits* you by putting the job in its proper, serious proportions. Primarily, this is presented as a diet plan for women. But by skipping the beauty hints, the same menus could work as effectively for men.

Most importantly, the imaginative recipes in this book prove that you *can* eat enjoyably while losing pounds. I find many of them unusually appealing. (Doctors eat too, you know.) Although low calorie, they are also balanced and varied enough to give you the nutritional values your body needs.

As a physician, I would add two suggestions. One, that it is important to take vitamins daily while dieting—one of the common all-inclusive compound vitamin supplements if you are 24 years of age or younger and a good B complex and C vitamin supplement if you are over that age. The other suggestion is a common-sense check with your doctor before undertaking the physical exercises recommended. For people in good shape, they should present no problems. But if you have (or have had) some type of ailment, your personal physician is best able to counsel you on what exercises are permissible for you.

In dealing with my own overweight patients, I always try to point out that there is more to eating than just eating. Diets go better when you make an event out of meals. To begin with, many of the recipes in this book involve more culinary effort than, say, just making a sandwich. You can anticipate how they will taste while going through the preparation. Then, try to arrange an attractive table because eye appeal is a big part of food enjoyment. Don't eat on the run or while standing in the kitchen. Eat slowly, savor each bite, and you'll be surprised how little it takes to abate hunger pangs.

Even though the author suggests you tear out each page and throw it away as the days progress, I think I'd keep some of the recipes on hand for future reference. They're that tasty, and the combination of dishes being both appetizing and low calorie at the same time is rather unusual in the tough world of weight losing.

In short, THE NO CHOICE DIET impresses me as a practical and psychologically oriented way to slim off a realistic amount of pounds. It doesn't prom-

A Foreword From A Physician

ise you the world, but it does incorporate many ingenious ideas on how to keep yourself in a dieting frame of mind. And that's a major part of the battle. Follow the schedule, step by step and day by day, and I think you will find that this diet *works*. Success, of course, is up to your perseverance. But when you find that you have lost those ugly pounds, you will realize that looking slimmer also means feeling fitter. Believe me, it's one of the best favors you can do for yourself.

I won't wish you good luck because successful dieting depends on a lot more than luck. Dieting is a state of mind. And it takes unwavering discipline to control how much of what you eat. This is a book that intelligently spells it all out for you. After all, being fit is infinitely more desirable than being fat.

JOHN PRUTTING, M.D.

Saturday

Today you should make all your physical preparations for beginning your diet on Monday. You may follow your normal routine for the day, but at some point you should do the following:

1. Weigh yourself. Write it on a sheet of paper. Subtract 10 pounds from it and write that next to it. Keep this paper in a prominent place.

2. Rid yourself of temptations. If you live alone, make a clean sweep of your cupboards and refrigerator. Throw out anything that could tempt you to stray off your diet: cookies, crackers, peanuts, pretzels, olives—anything that is not on the shopping list for Saturday. *Be ruthless.* Don't let a little penny-pinching keep you from dieting success. If you don't live alone, isolate everybody else's food from yours and mark off the division with a strip of masking tape. That single strip of tape is your demilitarized zone.

3. Check the shopping list to make sure you have on hand the spices and food staples you'll need for the diet recipes. Any you don't have, add to the shopping list. And *don't skimp.* These are critical items in making the delicious and varied new dishes you'll be preparing during the days ahead. It may cost you a few dollars, but this is the major food investment you'll be making for the next 33 days.

4. Shop for the foods you'll need for Week 1. The second part of Saturday's shopping contains all the foods you will need to carry you through next Saturday morning. One useful hint: Always do your food shopping after a meal. It's far easier to resist temptation when you're not hungry.

5. Buy one paperback book that you would like to read and a favorite magazine or two. These should be enjoyable (don't try to teach yourself French) and should have as little to do with food as possible.

6. Buy a vitamin-mineral supplement to be taken once a day.

7. Buy a 10-inch nonstick frying pan, if you don't already have one. Even when you're not on a diet, it will be useful in preparing many dishes in a healthful and nutritious way.

Shopping List

Herbs and spices
Basil (dried)
Bay leaves (whole, dried)
Cinnamon (ground)
Coriander (ground)
Cumin (ground)
Curry powder
Dill weed (dried)
Garlic salt
Ginger (ground)

Marjoram (dried)
Mint (dried)
Onion powder
Paprika
Peppercorns (whole, black)
Rosemary (dried)
Tarragon (dried)
Thyme (dried)

Condiments and flavorings
Capers
Horseradish
Prepared mustard
Poppy seeds
Sesame seeds
Soy sauce
Vanilla extract
Worcestershire sauce
Red pepper sauce

Saturday

Food staples

Bouillion cubes (beef, chicken, vegetable)

Parmesan cheese (grated)

Flour (unbleached, white)

Brown sugar

White sugar

Red wine vinegar

White vinegar

Herb tea bags (mint, rose hips, fruit blend, camomile, etc.)

Tea bags

Coffee

Decaffeinated instant coffee

Instant espresso coffee

Salt

Wheat germ (toasted)

Low-calorie Italian salad dressing

Low-calorie bleu-cheese salad dressing

Safflower oil

Peanut butter

Cornstarch

Breads

1 loaf cracked wheat bread

1 6-ounce box plain melba rounds

Dairy products

1 quart skim milk

1 12-ounce container cottage cheese

1 8-ounce container pineapple cottage cheese

1 8-ounce container plain yogurt

1 dozen medium eggs

Fruits and vegetables

1 3-inch apple

2 7-inch bananas

½ pound seedless green grapes

8 lemons

1 3-inch orange

1 quart orange juice

1 bag frozen unsweetened strawberries

2 2½-inch tangerines

1 4-inch grapefruit

1 3-inch pear

1 1-pound bag frozen cut green beans

1 bunch carrots

1 1-pint carton cherry tomatoes

1 12-ounce tomato juice

1 head garlic

1 head Boston lettuce

1 head iceberg lettuce

1 head romaine lettuce

½ pound medium mushrooms (about 16)

1 pound small new potatoes (6 to a pound)

1 pound baking potatoes (3 to a pound)

1 pound onions (4 to a pound)

1 bunch scallions

1 pound fresh spinach

1 bunch parsley

1 6-inch zucchini

Meat and fish

1 pound ground beef round

1 12-ounce chicken breast

¼ pound veal for scaloppine (store in freezer)

1 1-pound package frozen flounder fillets

1 1-pound bag frozen raw medium shrimp

1 4-ounce package sliced boiled ham (freeze remainder after use this week)

1 3½-ounce can solid white tuna (water-packed)

Other items

1 small jar olive oil

1 8-ounce package spaghetti

1 8-ounce jar diet or imitation mayonnaise

2 11-ounce bottles mineral water

Sunday

Today you can relax and enjoy yourself. You're about to do something you've been looking forward to for a long time: shed 10 ugly pounds. You should revel in the thought.

There are basic psychological preparations you can make that will reap big dividends in the days ahead. So some time during the day do the following:

1. Make a list of situations in which you find that you overeat: for example, watching television; at parties; when the office coffee wagon goes by; when you're upset or anxious. Put the list in a prominent place and add to it as new plights confront you. The program in the days ahead will offer help in coping with these situations. For now, remember two basic rules: (1) if you know you're going into a situation in which you normally indulge yourself (e.g., a party), have a small high-protein snack before you go (a square of cheese, a scoop of cottage cheese); (2) when the urge to eat hits you, do something else immediately. Read that paperback book you bought; go for a walk; take out the garbage.

2. Make a list of small household improvements you'd like to accomplish. They should be tasks that give you a sense of accomplishment and use up nervous energy. Clean out a closet; organize your photograph collection; refinish a bookcase; hang a few pictures. These tasks will divert your attention from food and provide you with a tremendous sense of satisfaction.

3. Telephone a friend and tell him or her about your diet. You will need friendly support along the way. Do not tell your skinny friend who is always muttering about how she would like to gain a few pounds. Do not tell your cousin who gives lectures on how easy it is to exert willpower. Tell only those people you know will be sympathetic.

Eating out

Eating out at a restaurant. If you have lunch in a restaurant, eat salad with a squeeze of lemon juice instead of dressing. If you cannot get a salad and decide to eat a complete meal, have baked or roasted chicken (without the skin); roast veal (without gravy); broiled or poached fish (cooked without fat). Augment with a fresh vegetable and a small baked potato with salt and pepper. Then, eat the lunch from the diet in the evening.

If you eat dinner out, follow the instructions above for the lunch. Make sure you choose a restaurant that can accommodate your needs.

Eating out at a friend's home. If you are very friendly with the host or hostess, tell him or her about your diet. If not, eat with care, avoiding gravies and sauces, bread and butter, and any condiments that are high in calories. If dessert is anything but fresh fruit, eat just a few spoonfuls to be polite. Do not use dining out as an excuse to overeat.

Reward yourself

When you have lost 3 pounds, give yourself a present. It should be a luxury—not necessarily expensive but something that makes you feel good and that you would not ordinarily buy. A record, a book, new eye makeup. When you have lost 5 pounds, give yourself another present. This one should be a good-looking piece of clothing in the size you will be when you lose the full 10 pounds (a 10-pound loss is one clothing size). When you have lost 8 pounds, give yourself *another* present. This one should be an appointment for a new hair style, a professional facial, a manicure or pedicure—a luxurious service that will make you look and feel better. When you have lost 10 pounds, you will have achieved your goal and you will feel great, but give yourself a present to celebrate your achievement. This should be something that you can wear or keep prominently displayed, which symbolizes your achievement. It could be a gold chain, a picture you love, or an interesting piece of sculpture.

Monday

Morning

On arising: **breathing exercise.** Start off each day with this deep-breathing exercise to be more alert and energetic. When you increase your oxygen intake, you wake up your whole system. Sit very tall on the edge of the bed with your feet planted firmly on the floor. Rest your hands on your thighs. Now, still keeping the spine erect, relax the stomach muscles; breathe in through the nose slowly and as deeply as possible. Your stomach should be forced outward like an inflated balloon. Keep taking short breaths until your lungs are full. When you have inhaled as deeply as you can, pause for a moment. Then slowly exhale, relaxing your chest and releasing air gradually. Tense your abdominal muscles to release even more air. Breathe in and out 10 times.

Immediately after breathing exercise: **wake-up exercises.** The vitality that comes from a brief morning workout is not only good in itself, it will help see you through the morning and make you less dependent on food. Start with the simple exercises below, and as you proceed with the diet, other exercises will be added.

Spine stretch

1. Stand with feet shoulder width apart. Lift arms straight up and then reach as high as you can with your right hand.

2. Relax right arm and reach as high as you can with your left hand. Repeat 10 times.

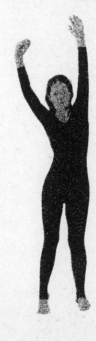

Running in place. Always run on a carpeted or padded surface. Warm up with a slow jog for 30 steps. Arms should be bent at elbows and held close to the body. Lift feet 3 or 4 inches off the floor. Imitate the heel-toe alternation of normal running. After you have warmed up, rest for a moment and then run at a faster pace, lifting legs and feet higher. Run for 1 minute. Cool down by walking around, taking big strides, until your pulse rate and breathing have returned to normal.

Weigh yourself and record your weight.

Note: In all menus, recipes are given for starred foods.

Breakfast menu (234 calories)
1 4-ounce glass orange juice (55 calories)
¼ cup pineapple cottage cheese, to use as spread on toast (70 calories)
1 slice cracked wheat toast (65 calories)
1 4-ounce glass skim milk (44 calories)
Coffee (regular or decaffeinated) or tea (no sugar)

Brown-bag lunch: If you are taking lunch to your office, prepare it right after breakfast.

"Whatever you can do, or dream you can, begin it.
Boldness has genius, power, and magic in it."
—GOETHE

Monday

Daytime

Midmorning break: **herb tea.**

Lunch menu (242 calories)
*Tossed salad with shrimp (119 calories)
*¼ cup tomato juice salad dressing (13 calories)
1 slice cracked wheat bread (65 calories)
½ apple (45 calories)

*Tossed salad with shrimp
10 boiled shrimp (100 calories)
2 cups Boston and romaine lettuce, torn   into bite-sized pieces (15 calories)
1 scallion, finely chopped (4 calories)

Combine shrimp, lettuce, and scallion. Toss to mix thoroughly. Drizzle dressing over all immediately before serving.

*Tomato juice salad dressing
½ cup tomato juice (23 calories)
1 tablespoon lemon juice (3 calories)
½ teaspoon prepared horseradish
1 dash Worcestershire sauce
¼ teaspoon onion powder
¼ teaspoon black pepper, freshly ground

Combine all ingredients in a cup and stir until well blended. Refrigerate remaining dressing to use for dinner on Day 2.

Midafternoon break: The midafternoon slump that almost everyone experiences can be eliminated with a simple exercise break. This consists of a minute of running in place. If you are at work, go to a lounge and do your running there. If that isn't possible, walk very briskly for several minutes. You will find this a stimulating pickup, and it adds no calories at all.

Evening

Dinner menu (513 calories)
*½ herb-lemon baked chicken breast (145 calories)
3 sliced carrots, steamed (50 calories) and sprinkled with 1
   tablespoon chopped parsley (2 calories)
*Spinach and mushroom salad (51 calories)
*1 tablespoon lemon-cumin salad dressing (50 calories)
1 orange, peeled and sliced (64 calories) and 1 banana, sliced (80
   calories), combined with ¼ cup orange juice (27 calories)
*Cappuccino (made with ½ cup instant espresso and ½ cup hot skim mil¹
   sprinkled with cinnamon) (44 calories)

*Herb-lemon baked chicken breast

1 12-ounce chicken breast, cut in half (288 calories)	½ teaspoon tarragon
	½ teaspoon onion powder
2 tablespoons lemon juice (6 calories)	½ teaspoon salt
½ teaspoon thyme	½ teaspoon black pepper, freshly ground

Marinate chicken pieces in lemon juice for about 30 minutes. Place chicken breast in baking pan. Sprinkle with herbs and other seasonings. Bake uncovered in 400° oven for 45 minutes. Use ½ for lunch on Day 2. (Calorie counts for marinated foods are based on ½ of the marinade contributing calories to the dish.)

*Spinach and mushroom salad

¼ pound fresh spinach leaves, stems removed (22 calories)	5 mushrooms, sliced (25 calories)
	1 scallion, finely chopped (4 calories)

Wash spinach leaves thoroughly, dry on paper towels, and tear into bite-sized pieces. Combine spinach with mushrooms (wiped with a damp paper towel and sliced). Sprinkle with chopped scallion. Just before serving, add lemon-cumin salad dressing.

*Lemon-cumin salad dressing (use on subsequent days)
(1005 calories, approximately 50 calories per tablespoon)

½ cup safflower or other polyunsaturated oil (972 calories)	1 clove garlic, finely minced (optional) (3 calories)
½ cup lemon juice (30 calories)	½ teaspoon salt
¼ cup water	¼ teaspoon black pepper, freshly ground
¼ teaspoon cumin	

Combine all ingredients and mix in blender. Use 1 tablespoon per serving. Refrigerate to store and shake before using.

Eleven o'clock exercise break: mat exercises to relax you and tone your muscles. Before retiring, do the firming exercises below. If you schedule them right after the late evening news, you'll find they can become a nightly habit.

Knee lift

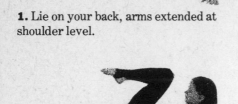

1. Lie on your back, arms extended at shoulder level.

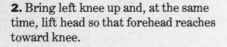

2. Bring left knee up and, at the same time, lift head so that forehead reaches toward knee.

3. Repeat with right knee. Alternate knees, bringing each knee up 10 times.

Crisscross

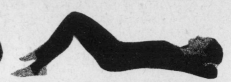

1. Lie on your back, hands clasped behind your head. Have knees bent and feet flat on floor.

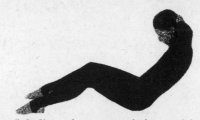

2. Inhaling, rise up to a sitting position.

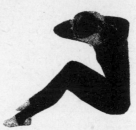

3. Touch right elbow to left knee. Exhaling, slowly lie down.

4. Repeat, touching left elbow to right knee. Alternate 10 times.

Last thing before you go to bed: **nature meditation.** This relaxing exercise helps to induce sleep. Read it all the way through before you begin.

Lie on your back on a mat, legs slightly separated and arms at your sides, palms of hands facing up. Imagine a summer day in a pine woods. As you walk along a footpath, streaks of sunlight pierce the trees overhead. A lake glitters in the distance. There is a large, smooth rock at the water's edge, and you sit down to watch the sunlight playing on the incredibly clear water. Birds call to each other. There is a strong fragrance of pine. A deer comes to drink at the opposite edge of the lake. Let yourself savor the peacefulness of the scene. When you are restful and serene, you are ready for a good night's sleep.

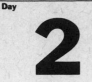

Morning

On arising: **breathing exercise.** Sit very tall on the edge of the bed with your feet planted firmly on the floor. Rest your hands on your thighs. Now, still keeping your spine erect, relax stomach muscles; breathe in slowly and as deeply as possible. Your stomach should be forced outward like an inflated balloon. Keep taking short breaths until your lungs are full. When you have breathed in as fully as you can, pause for a moment. Then slowly exhale, relaxing your chest and releasing air gradually. Tense your abdominal muscles to release even more air. Breathe in and out 10 times.

Immediately after breathing exercise: **wake-up exercises.** The vitality that comes from a brief morning workout is not only good in itself, it will help see you through the morning and make you less dependent on food.

Arm circles

1. Stand with feet shoulder width apart. Raise arms to shoulder height. Moving arms forward, make 10 circles in the air.

2. Reverse direction and make 10 more circles.

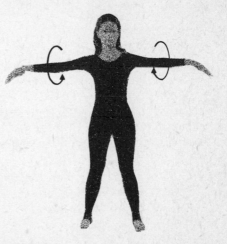

Running in place. Always run on a carpeted or padded surface. Warm up with a slow jog for 30 steps. Arms should be bent at elbows and held close to the body. Lift feet 3 or 4 inches off the floor. Imitate the heel-toe alternation of normal running. After you have warmed up, rest for a moment and then run at a faster pace, lifting legs and feet higher. Run for 1 minute. Cool down by walking around, taking big strides, until your pulse rate and breathing have returned to normal.

Weigh yourself and record your weight.

Breakfast menu (242 calories)
1 4-ounce glass orange juice (55 calories)
1 egg, poached (78 calories)
1 slice cracked wheat toast (65 calories)
1 4-ounce glass skim milk (44 calories)
Coffee (regular or decaffeinated) or tea (no sugar)

Brown-bag lunch: If you are taking lunch to your office, prepare it right after breakfast.

Tuesday

Daytime

Midmorning break: **herb tea.**

Lunch menu (288 calories)
*Chicken salad (208 calories)
1 carrot, cut into sticks (17 calories)
3 melba toast rounds (24 calories)
1 tangerine (39 calories)
Coffee (regular or decaffeinated) or tea (no sugar or milk)

*Chicken salad
½ herb-lemon baked chicken breast, skinned, boned, and diced (from Day 1) (145 calories)
1 tablespoon diet or imitation mayonnaise (48 calories)
1 teaspoon lemon juice (1 calorie)
1 dash red pepper sauce
1 scallion, thinly sliced (4 calories)
¼ head iceberg lettuce, shredded (10 calories)

Combine chicken, mayonnaise, lemon juice, pepper sauce, and scallion. Mix thoroughly. Serve on shredded iceberg lettuce.

Midafternoon break: Run in place for 1 minute. After you cool down, eat ½ banana (40 calories).

Beauty break checklist for upcoming week
Loofah sponge
Castile soap
Scented body lotion
Mild soap
Dried mint
1 8-ounce container yogurt
Moisturizer
pH-balanced protein shampoo
Protein hair conditioner
Wide-toothed comb

Tuesday

Evening

Dinner menu (471 calories)

1 11-ounce glass mineral water with ice and a thin slice of lemon
*1 3-ounce grilled seasoned hamburger (188 calories)
*1 baked potato (90 calories)
1 zucchini, steamed (26 calories) and sprinkled with 1 chopped scallion
    (4 calories) and 1 tablespoon lemon juice (1 calorie)
Tossed green salad made from ¼ head iceberg lettuce, shredded (10 calories),
    3 cherry tomatoes, halved (12 calories), and 1 tablespoon chopped parsley
    (2 calories); serve with 1 tablespoon tomato juice salad dressing (3 calories)
*¼ cup cottage cheese "sour cream" with green grapes (135 calories)

*Grilled seasoned hamburger

1 pound ground beef round; shape into 3 3-ounce hamburgers and 4 small meatballs. Freeze 1 hamburger patty and the meatballs. (1,008 calories)	¼ teaspoon black pepper 1 tablespoon Worcestershire sauce 1 teaspoon onion powder ¼ teaspoon garlic powder
1 teaspoon salt	

Broil the 2 hamburgers 4 inches from flame to desired doneness and remove from broiler. Refrigerate 1 patty to be served as sliced meatloaf for lunch on Day 3.

*Baked potato

Bake a well-washed potato for 40 minutes in a 400° oven; reduce heat to 350° and bake for 10 minutes more. Prick the skin of the potato with a fork about halfway through cooking time. To serve, split open with a knife and sprinkle with salt, pepper, and paprika.

*Cottage cheese "sour cream" with green grapes

¼ cup cottage cheese (60 calories)	½ cup green grapes (50 calories)
1 to 2 tablespoons skim milk (11 calories)	1 teaspoon brown sugar (14 calories)

To make cottage cheese "sour cream" (which has half the calories of regular sour cream) put cottage cheese and skim milk in container of blender and whir until smooth and creamy. Combine grapes and "sour cream." Sprinkle with brown sugar.

Eleven o'clock exercise break: mat exercises to relax you and tone your muscles.

Leg up and over

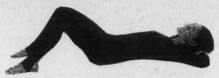

Crisscross

1. Lie on your back, hands clasped behind your head. Have knees bent and feet flat on floor.

1. Lie on your back, arms extended at shoulder level. Bend right knee.

2. Straighten leg up into air, toes pointed. Hold for a count of 3.

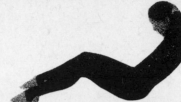

2. Inhaling, rise up to a sitting position.

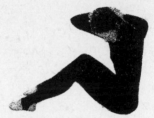

3. Swing leg over to touch floor on left side as close to left hand as possible. Keep arms and head stationary. Swing leg back to center and lower. Repeat with left leg. Do each leg 5 times.

3. Touch right elbow to left knee. Exhaling, slowly lie down.

4. Repeat, touching left elbow to right knee. Alternate 10 times.

Beauty break: **loofah sponge beauty bath.** A loofah is a vegetable sponge made from a special variety of gourd. When a loofah is softened in water it has just the right texture to cleanse the body skin of dead cells and to stimulate circulation. Here is the best method of using a loofah effectively.

You will need: loofah sponge, castile soap, and scented body lotion.

Soak yourself and a loofah in a tub of warm water for about 5 minutes. Then rub the loofah against a cake of castile soap, working up a good lather. Using a vigorous circular motion, massage the skin of elbows, knees, and feet. When you move to more sensitive areas, such as the legs, arms, stomach, use a gentler touch. Reapply soap and go back over feet (especially the heels and soles), knees, and elbows. Rinse thoroughly. Step out of tub and then give yourself a brisk towel rubdown. Leave your skin slightly damp. Apply scented body lotion all over.

Morning

On arising: **breathing exercise.** Sit very tall on the edge of the bed with feet planted firmly on the floor. Rest your hands on your thighs. Now, still keeping your spine erect, relax stomach muscles; breathe in slowly and as deeply as possible. Your stomach should be forced outward like an inflated balloon. Keep taking short breaths until your lungs are full. When you have breathed in as fully as you can, pause for a moment. Then slowly exhale, relaxing your chest and releasing air gradually. Tense your abdominal muscles to release even more air. Breathe in and out 10 times.

Immediately after breathing exercise: **wake-up exercises.** Remember, these give you vitality and help make you less dependent on food.

Side stretch

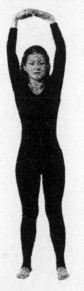
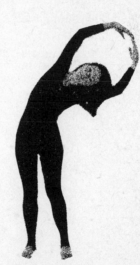

1. Stand with feet 6 inches apart. Breathe in deeply as you lift arms above head, placing one hand over the other.

2. Exhaling, bend to the left as far as is comfortable.

3. Go back to the center, breathing in. As you exhale, bend to the right as far as is comfortable. Stretch 10 times to each side.

Running in place. Always run on a carpeted or padded surface. Warm up with a slow jog for 30 steps. Arms should be bent at elbows and held close to the body. Lift feet 3 or 4 inches off the floor. Imitate the heel-toe alternation of normal running. After you have warmed up, rest for a moment and then run at a faster pace, lifting legs and feet higher. Run for 1 minute. Cool down by walking around, taking big strides, until your pulse rate and breathing have returned to normal.

Weigh yourself and record your weight.

Breakfast menu (224 calories)
1 4-ounce glass orange juice (55 calories)
¼ cup cottage cheese, sprinkled with cinnamon, to use as spread for toast (60 calories)
1 slice cracked wheat toast (65 calories)
1 4-ounce glass skim milk (44 calories)
Coffee (regular or decaffeinated) or tea (no sugar)

Brown-bag lunch: If you are taking lunch to your office, prepare it right after breakfast.

Note: Transfer frozen flounder fillets from freezer to refrigerator.

"A good meal ought to begin with hunger."
—FRENCH PROVERB

3 | Wednesday

Daytime

Midmorning break: **herb tea.**

Lunch menu (284 calories)
1 grilled seasoned hamburger, chilled and sliced from dinner on Day 2 (188 calories)
1 teaspoon mustard (8 calories)
4 melba toast rounds (32 calories)
4 cherry tomatoes (16 calories)
½ banana (40 calories)
Coffee (regular or decaffeinated) or tea (no sugar or milk)

Midafternoon break: Run in place for 1 minute. After cooling off, slowly sip a cup of hot vegetable broth.

Wednesday

Evening

Dinner menu (423 calories)

*Baked flounder fillets Provençal (143 calories)

3 new potatoes, boiled (90 calories)

Tossed green salad made from ¼ head romaine lettuce, torn into bite-sized pieces (10 calories); serve with 1 tablespoon lemon-cumin salad dressing (50 calories)

1 pear (95 calories) cut in half, cored, and filled with 2 tablespoons pineapple cottage cheese (35 calories)

Coffee (regular or decaffenated) or tea (no sugar)

*Baked flounder fillets Provençal

4 ounces flounder fillets (fresh, or thawed only enough to separate pieces) (79 calories)

Sauce:

½ can (4 ounces) tomato sauce (40 calories)

½ onion, finely chopped (19 calories)

1 clove garlic, minced (3 calories)

¼ teaspoon thyme

½ bay leaf

1 tablespoon fresh parsley, finely chopped (2 calories)

¼ cup water

Into a small saucepan put the tomato sauce, onion, garlic, herbs, and water. Simmer for 15 minutes. Place fillets in small baking dish and cover with sauce. Bake in a 300° oven for 15 minutes.

Eleven o'clock exercise break: mat exercises to relax you and tone your muscles.

Knee and head lifts

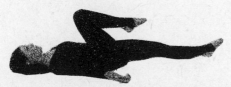

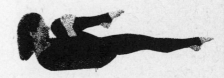

1. Lie on your back, arms at sides, palms down. Bend right knee and pull toward chest.

2. Inhaling, grasp leg with hands just below knee. At the same time, raise head and touch forehead to knee. Exhaling, return to starting position. Repeat 10 times.

Leg up and over

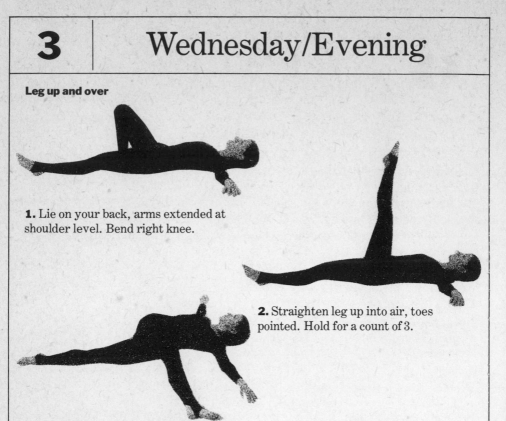

1. Lie on your back, arms extended at shoulder level. Bend right knee.

2. Straighten leg up into air, toes pointed. Hold for a count of 3.

3. Swing leg over to touch floor on left side as close to left hand as possible. Keep arms and head stationary. Swing leg back to center and lower. Repeat with left leg. Do each leg 5 times.

Last thing before going to bed: **color meditation.** This is another relaxing exercise that eliminates tensions and encourages sleep. Read instructions all the way through before you begin.

Lie on your back on a mat, with your legs slightly separated and relaxed and your arms at your sides, palms facing up. Think of your favorite color. Imagine beautiful clothes in this color. Dress yourself in them. Next, imagine you are painting a room, quickly and effortlessly, in a beautiful shade of your favorite color. A large cushion of the same shade is the only furnishing. Sit on the cushion and let yourself savor the pleasure of being surrounded by the beautiful color.

Morning

On arising: **breathing exercise.** Sit very tall on the edge of the bed with your feet planted firmly on the floor. Rest your hands on your thighs. Now, still keeping your spine erect, relax stomach muscles; breathe in slowly and as deeply as possible. Your stomach should be forced outward like an inflated balloon. Keep taking short breaths until your lungs are full. When you have breathed in as fully as you can, pause for a moment. Then slowly exhale, relaxing your chest and releasing air gradually. Tense your abdominal muscles to release even more air. Breathe in and out 12 times.

Immediately after breathing exercises: **wake-up exercises.** Don't forget these give you vitality and will help make you less dependent on food.

Overhead arm swing

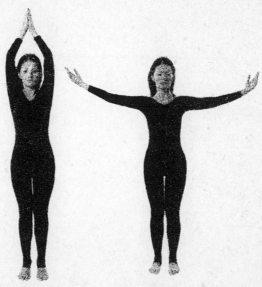

1. Stand with feet together. Lift up on toes, breathing in and raising arms until palms meet overhead.

2. Breathe out as you lower heels to floor and bring arms down to your sides. Repeat 10 times.

Running in place. Always run on a carpeted or padded surface. Warm up with a slow jog for 30 steps. Arms should be bent at elbows and held close to the body. Lift feet 3 or 4 inches off the floor. Imitate the heel-toe alternation of normal running. After you have warmed up, rest for a moment and then run at a faster pace, lifting the legs and feet higher. Run for 1½ minutes. Cool down by walking around, taking big strides, until your pulse rate and breathing have returned to normal.

Weigh yourself and record your weight.

Breakfast menu (235 calories)
½ grapefruit (48 calories)
1 egg, fried in nonstick pan (78 calories)
1 slice cracked wheat toast (65 calories)
1 4-ounce glass skim milk (44 calories)
Coffee (regular or decaffeinated) or tea (no sugar)

Brown-bag lunch: If you are taking lunch to your office, prepare it right after breakfast.

Note: Transfer veal from freezer to refrigerator.

"He who has begun has half done."
—HORACE

Daytime

Midmorning break: **herb tea.**

Lunch menu (266 calories)
*Open-faced tuna salad sandwich (227 calories)
1 tangerine (39 calories)
Coffee (regular or decaffeinated) or tea (no sugar or milk)

*Open-faced tuna salad sandwich
1 3½-ounce can solid white tuna, water-packed (120 calories)
1 teaspoon capers (3 calories)
1 scallion, finely chopped (4 calories)
1 teaspoon lemon juice (1 calorie)

2 teaspoons imitation or diet mayonnaise (32 calories)
1 leaf romaine lettuce (2 calories)
1 slice cracked wheat bread (65 calories)

Combine drained tuna, capers, scallion, lemon juice, and mayonnaise and mix thoroughly. Tear romaine lettuce leaf into small pieces. Cover bread with lettuce, then with the tuna salad.

Midafternoon break: Run in place for 1 minute. After cooling off, have a cup of herb tea.

Evening

Dinner menu (480 calories)
*Veal scaloppine with lemon and mushrooms (350 calories)

1 cup green beans, steamed and sprinkled with a pinch of dried or fresh dill weed (40 calories)

Tossed green salad made from ¼ head romaine lettuce, torn into bite-sized pieces (10 calories); serve with 1 tablespoon low-calorie Italian salad dressing (7 calories)

½ apple, cored and sliced (45 calories), dipped in cinnamon-and-sugar mix (½ teaspoon cinnamon mixed with 2 teaspoons sugar) (28 calories)

Instant espresso with lemon peel, coffee (regular or decaffeinated) or tea (no sugar or milk)

*Veal scaloppine with lemon and mushrooms

4 ounces veal for scallopine (247 calories)	1 tablespoon lemon juice (3 calories)
1 teaspoon flour (9 calories)	¼ cup chicken broth, made from bouillon cube (1 calorie)
2 teaspoons olive oil (66 calories)	
5 mushrooms (25 calories)	Salt and pepper
¼ teaspoon marjoram	1 teaspoon parsley, chopped

Dust veal lightly with flour. Brown slices in olive oil in nonstick pan. Remove veal and add sliced mushrooms, lemon juice, broth, herbs, salt, and pepper. Cook for 5 minutes over medium heat. Add veal, cook for 1 or 2 minutes. Sprinkle with parsley and serve.

Beauty break: **home facial.** Giving yourself a facial, one that really cleans and tones your skin, is easy. Make it a once-a-month part of your beauty program.

You will need: mild soap, 2-quart saucepan filled with 1 quart water, 1 teaspoon dried mint, 1 towel, ½ container plain yogurt, and moisturizer.

Bring water to a boil and add dried mint. Remove from stove and set on a heat-proof steady table. In the meantime, tie or pin hair back, away from face. Work up a lather with soap and wash your face thoroughly. Rinse with warm water. While liquid in pot is still steaming *(test with your hand to see that it is not too hot),* hold your face about a foot above the pot. Cover your head with a towel that reaches down to cover the pot. Remember, steam should be comfortably warm—not hot. After the warm moisture has opened the pores, apply the cold yogurt to your face. Lie down on a bed with your feet elevated until the yogurt dries. Rinse off with several splashings of warm water. Dry face lightly with a towel and then apply a thin layer of moisturizer to your still slightly damp skin.

Eleven o'clock exercise break: mat exercises to relax you and tone your muscles.

Sitbacks

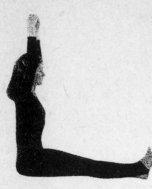

1. Sit with legs together straight out in front of you. Lift arms straight up.

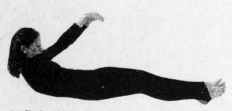

2. Lower head and arms, contract stomach muscles, and roll back slowly.

3. Go back until shoulders almost touch floor. Slowly return to starting position. Repeat 5 times.

Knee and head lifts

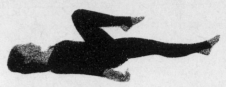

1. Lie on your back, arms at sides, palms down. Bend right knee and pull toward chest.

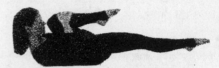

2. Inhaling, grasp leg with hands just below knee. At the same time, raise head and touch forehead to knee. Exhaling, return to starting position. Repeat 10 times.

Friday

Morning

On arising: **breathing exercise.** Sit very tall on the edge of the bed with your feet planted firmly on the floor. Rest your hands on your thighs. Now, still keeping your spine erect, relax stomach muscles; breathe in slowly and as deeply as possible. Your stomach should be forced outward like an inflated balloon. Keep taking short breaths until your lungs are full. When you have breathed in as fully as you can, pause for a moment. Then slowly exhale, relaxing your chest and releasing air gradually. Tense your abdominal muscles to release even more air. Breathe in and out 12 times.

Immediately after breathing exercises: **wake-up exercises.**

Shoulder swing

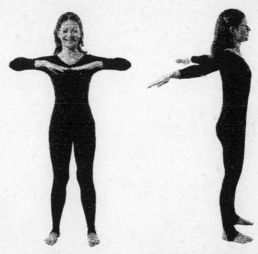

1. Stand with feet shoulder width apart. Raise arms to shoulder level, bend elbows, and bring arms close to chest.

2. Push elbows back. Open arms and bring hands back as far as is comfortable. Swing arms forward and back.

3. Fold arms back into chest. Move elbows back and forward twice. Return to starting position. Repeat 5 times.

5 | Friday/Morning

Running in place. Always run on a carpeted or padded surface. Warm up with a slow jog for 30 steps. Arms should be bent at elbows and held close to the body. Lift feet 3 or 4 inches off the floor. Imitate the heel-toe alternation of normal running. After you have warmed up, rest for a moment and then run at a faster pace, lifting the legs and feet higher. Run for 1½ minutes. Cool down by walking around, taking big strides, until your pulse rate and breathing have returned to normal.

Weigh yourself and record your weight.

Breakfast menu (217 calories)
½ grapefruit (48 calories)
¼ cup cottage cheese, sprinkled with cinnamon, to use as spread on toast (60 calories)
1 slice cracked wheat toast (65 calories)
1 4-ounce glass skim milk (44 calories)
Coffee (regular or decaffeinated) or tea (no sugar)

Brown-bag lunch: If you are taking lunch to your office, prepare it right after breakfast.

Note: Transfer frozen meatballs from freezer to refrigerator.

Friday

Daytime

Midmorning break: **herb tea.**

Lunch menu (250 calories)
*Spinach and egg salad (176 calories)
3 melba toast rounds (24 calories)
½ cup green grapes (50 calories)
Coffee (regular or decaffeinated) or tea (no sugar or milk)

*Spinach and egg salad
½ pound fresh spinach, washed, dried,
  and stems removed (44 calories)
1 hard-cooked egg, sliced (78 calories)
4 mushrooms, sliced (20 calories)

4 cherry tomatoes (16 calories)
1 scallion, finely chopped (4 calories)
2 tablespoons low-calorie Italian salad
  dressing (14 calories)

Hard-cook egg by putting it into cold water and bringing to a boil. Lower heat and simmer for 6 minutes; then turn off heat and let egg stand for 15 minutes. Tear spinach into bite-sized pieces. Combine all ingredients. Toss immediately before serving with salad dressing.

Midafternoon break: Run in place for 1 minute. After cooling off, have a cup of herb tea.

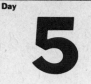
Friday

Evening

Note: If you plan to be out late on Friday evening, do mat exercises before dinner. Follow with relaxation technique.

Dinner menu (585 calories)
*Meatballs and spaghetti (469 calories), sprinkled with 1 tablespoon grated Parmesan cheese (20 calories)

Tossed green salad made from ¼ head romaine lettuce, torn into bite-sized pieces (10 calories); serve with 1 tablespoon low-calorie Italian salad dressing (7 calories)

1 cup strawberries (52 calories) with ¼ cup fresh orange juice (27 calories)

Instant espresso with lemon peel, coffee (regular or decaffeinated) or tea (no sugar or milk)

*Meatballs in sauce
2 meatballs (1¾ ounces each) thawed and browned in 400° oven for 20 minutes (219 calories)

Sauce:

1 teaspoon olive oil (33 calories)
½ can (4 ounces) tomato sauce
  (40 calories)
½ onion, finely chopped (19 calories)

1 clove garlic, minced (3 calories)
¼ teaspoon basil
Pinch of oregano

Combine all ingredients in small frying pan and simmer for 20 minutes over low heat. Add 2 tablespoons water to sauce as it thickens. Serve meatballs in sauce over spaghetti.

Spaghetti
For 1 cup cooked spaghetti, boil 3 ounces raw according to package directions. (155 calories)

Eleven o'clock exercise break: mat exercises to relax you and tone your muscles.

Sitbacks

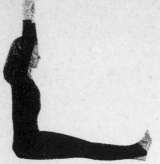

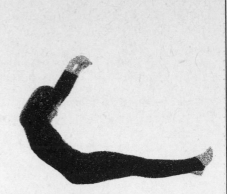

1. Sit with legs together straight out in front of you. Lift arms straight up.

2. Lower head and arms, contract stomach muscles, and roll back slowly.

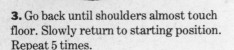

3. Go back until shoulders almost touch floor. Slowly return to starting position. Repeat 5 times.

Last thing before you go to bed: **the tense-and-relaxation technique.** This is a method of relaxation borrowed from hatha yoga. It is amazingly effective. Read instructions all the way through before you begin.

Lie on your back on a mat, with feet slightly apart, arms at your side and palms of hands facing up. Start the exercise by thinking of your toes and feet. Tense them as tightly as you can and then release the tension. Next, tense your right leg and release the tension. Do the same with your left leg. Tense your right arm, clenching your fist, and then release the tension. Repeat with the left arm and fist. Tense your shoulders and release the tension. Squeeze your lips, eyes, and face together, as though you were going to form a point, and release. Going back to your toes, think about relaxing each toe, the feet, the lower legs, thighs, buttocks, arms, back, the shoulders, the face and scalp, and the back of your neck. Consciously relax every part of your body by letting your soothing thoughts travel up and down.

Morning

On arising: **breathing exercise.** Sit very tall on the edge of the bed with your feet planted firmly on the floor. Rest your hands on your thighs. Now, still keeping your spine erect, relax stomach muscles; breathe in slowly and as deeply as possible. Your stomach should be forced outward like an inflated balloon. Keep taking short breaths until your lungs are full. When you have breathed in as fully as you can, pause for a moment. Then slowly exhale, relaxing your chest and releasing air gradually. Tense your abdominal muscles to release even more air. Breathe in and out 12 times.

Immediately after breathing exercises: **wake-up exercises.**

Spine stretch

1. Stand with feet shoulder width apart. Lift arms straight up and then reach as high as you can with your right hand.

2. Relax right arm and reach as high as you can with your left hand. Repeat 10 times.

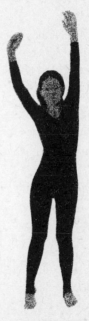

Running in place. Always run on a carpeted or padded surface. Warm up with a slow jog for 30 steps. Arms should be bent at elbows and held close to the body. Lift feet 3 or 4 inches off the floor. Imitate the heel-toe alternation of normal running. After you have warmed up, rest for a moment and then run at a faster pace, lifting the legs and feet higher. Run for 1½ minutes. Cool down by walking around, taking big strides, until your pulse rate and breathing have returned to normal.

Weigh yourself and record your weight.

Breakfast menu (263 calories)

1 4-ounce glass tomato juice, seasoned with a squeeze of lemon juice, dash Worcestershire sauce, and dash red pepper sauce (23 calories)
1 egg, poached (78 calories)
1 1-ounce slice lean boiled ham, heated in nonstick frying pan (53 calories)
1 slice cracked wheat toast (65 calories)
1 4-ounce glass skim milk (44 calories)
Coffee (regular or decaffeinated) or tea (no sugar)

Shopping List

Breads

1 package breadsticks (12 inches long)

Dairy products

1 quart skim milk
1 8-ounce container vanilla yogurt
1 8-ounce container coffee yogurt
1 6-ounce package sliced Swiss cheese
   (4 1½-ounce slices)

Fruits and vegetables

1 20-ounce jar unsweetened applesauce
1 3-inch apple
2 7-inch bananas
½ pound seedless green grapes
1 4-inch grapefruit
4 lemons
1 3-inch orange
1 2½-inch tangerine
1 3-inch pear
1 bunch broccoli (6 stalks)
1 7-inch cucumber
1 small fresh ginger root (if
unavailable, use ground ginger)
1 head Boston lettuce
1 head iceberg lettuce
1 head romaine lettuce
¼ pound medium mushrooms (about 8)
1 bunch parsley
1 1-pound bag frozen green peas

1 bunch scallions
½ pound spinach
1 12-ounce acorn squash

Meat and fish

2 12-ounce chicken breasts (store one in freezer)
¼ pound ham steak
¼ pound ground veal
¼ pound flank steak (store in freezer)
1 1-pound bag frozen raw medium shrimp
3 3½-ounce can solid white tuna, water-packed

Other items

1 8-ounce can roasted, slivered almonds
1 stick corn oil margarine
1 package bran flakes
3 11-ounce bottles mineral water

Daytime

Lunch menu (264 calories)
*Tuna salad (192 calories)
3 melba toast rounds (24 calories)
½ pear (48 calories)
Coffee (regular or decaffeinated) or tea (no sugar)

*Tuna Salad

1 3½-ounce can solid white tuna,
  water-packed (120 calories)
¼ head romaine lettuce, torn into
  bite-sized pieces (10 calories)

2 cherry tomatoes, halved (8 calories)
1 scallion, thinly sliced (4 calories)
1 tablespoon lemon-cumin salad dressing
  (50 calories)

Toss all ingredients together and mix thoroughly.

Note: Freeze ½ cup vanilla yogurt for dinner dessert. Remove an hour or more before serving.

Beauty break: **conditioning hair treatment and shampoo.** Make a conditioning treatment a once-a-week step in your beauty program, and your hair will always be silky, shiny, and easy to manage. Use a protein shampoo to wash hair before applying conditioner.

You will need: pH-balanced protein shampoo, protein conditioner, and a wide-toothed comb.

Wet hair under warm shower. Apply shampoo and work up a rich lather. Rinse thoroughly. Apply protein conditioner as directed on package. Comb conditioner through hair several times. Allow conditioner to remain on hair 20 minutes. Rinse conditioner out with luke-warm water. Blow-dry hair or let it dry naturally. If you have been using rollers or blow-drying your hair for years, try letting it dry naturally and use fingers to style hair. Natural hair styles are terrific looking and the most comfortable.

Beauty break checklist for upcoming week

Lipstick brush
Plum or rosy-brown lipstick
Pink-beige lipstick
Clear lip gloss
Magnifying mirror
Cotton pads
Nail clippers
Orangewood stick

Nail polish
Nail polish remover
Nail finish coat
Moisturizer
Mild soap
2 makeup sponges
Toning lotion
Lightweight makeup foundation
Blusher

Evening

Dinner menu (509 calories)

1 11-ounce glass mineral water with ice and a thin slice of lemon
*Lemon-garlic shrimp (179 calories)
Rice and peas made with ½ cup cooked white rice (112 calories) mixed with
   ½ cup cooked green peas (68 calories)
Tossed green salad made from 2 cups romaine and Boston lettuce leaves,
   torn into bite-sized pieces (15 calories) and 1 tablespoon chopped parsley
   (2 calories); serve with 1 tablespoon tomato juice salad dressing
   (7 calories)
Frozen vanilla yogurt with strawberries made with ½ cup vanilla yogurt
   (100 calories) frozen for several hours in the freezer and mixed with ½ cup
   fresh or slightly thawed, unsweetened strawberries (26 calories)
Instant espresso with small strip of lemon peel, coffee (regular or
   decaffeinated), or tea (no sugar or milk)

*Lemon-garlic shrimp

10 raw shrimp (100 calories)
2 teaspoons margarine (67 calories)
1 clove garlic, minced (3 calories)
2 tablespoons lemon juice (6 calories)

¼ cup chicken stock, made from chicken
   bouillon cube (1 calorie)
1 tablespoon parsley, minced (2 calories)

Melt margarine in small frying pan over medium-high heat. Add garlic and sauté for 1 minute. Add lemon juice and chicken stock and bring to a boil. Continue cooking for several minutes. Add the shrimp and cook until shrimp turns pink. Turn and cook on the other side for 2 or 3 minutes. Sprinkle parsley over shrimp and cook for 1 minute more.

Eleven o'clock exercise break: mat exercises to relax you and tone your muscles.

Pelvic twist

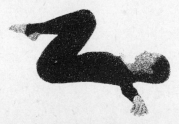 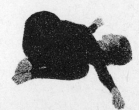

1. Lie on your back, arms out at shoulder level. Inhaling, raise both knees and bring as close to body as possible.

2. Exhaling, roll to the right so that right knee and ankle touch floor. Roll over to the left, touching floor. Roll to each side 5 times.

Morning

On arising: **breathing exercise.** Sit very tall on the edge of the bed with your feet planted firmly on the floor. Rest your hands on your thighs. Now, keeping your spine erect, relax stomach muscles and inhale slowly, as deeply as possible. Your abdomen should be forced outward like an inflated balloon. Take short breaths until your lungs are filled. When you have inhaled to capacity, pause for a moment. Then slowly exhale, relaxing your chest and releasing air gradually. Tighten your abdominal muscles to expel even more air. Repeat this exercise 12 times.

Immediately after breathing exercise: **wake-up exercises.**

Weigh yourself and record your weight.

No running in place on Sundays.

Shoulder swing

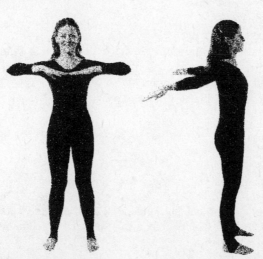

1. Stand with feet shoulder width apart. Raise arms to shoulder level, bend elbows, and bring arms close to chest.

2. Push elbows back. Open arms and bring hands back as far as is comfortable. Swing arms forward and back.

3. Fold arms back into chest. Move elbows back and forward twice. Return to starting position. Repeat 5 times.

Spine stretch

1. Stand with feet shoulder width apart. Lift arms straight up and then reach as high as you can with your right hand.

2. Relax right arm and reach as high as you can with your left hand. Repeat 10 times.

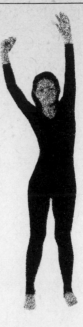

Breakfast menu (344 calories)

1 4-ounce glass orange juice (55 calories)
*2 slices French toast (190 calories)
½ cup unsweetened applesauce, mixed with ½ teaspoon cinnamon
(55 calories)
1 4-ounce glass skim milk (44 calories)
Coffee (regular or decaffeinated) or tea (no sugar)

*French toast

1 egg (78 calories)
½ cup skim milk (44 calories)
½ teaspoon vanilla extract

4 slices cracked wheat bread (65 calories per slice)

Combine egg with skim milk and vanilla. Beat vigorously with a rotary beater. Dip slice of bread in egg mixture. There will be enough for 4 slices of French toast. Cook all 4 slices in a nonstick frying pan until golden, 2 for today and 2 wrapped individually in foil, to freeze for later use. Serve 2 slices spread with cinnamon applesauce.

Sunday

Daytime

Lunch menu (250 calories)
*Grilled Swiss cheese sandwich (171 calories)
Tossed green salad made from ¼ head iceberg lettuce, shredded (10 calories) and 3 cherry tomatoes, halved (12 calories); serve with 1 tablespoon low-calorie Italian salad dressing (7 calories)
½ cup green grapes (50 calories)
Coffee (regular or decaffeinated) or tea (no sugar or milk)

*Grilled Swiss cheese sandwich
1 1-ounce slice Swiss cheese (106 calories)
1 slice cracked wheat bread (65 calories)

Lightly toast bread in toaster. Place cheese on toast and place under broiler until cheese melts.

Midafternoon break: **a brisk 2-mile walk.** Choose a destination a mile distant, one that you will enjoy—a museum, garden, river, local monument. Walk there and back at a brisk pace. On returning home, relax with a cup of herb tea.

7 | Sunday

Evening

Dinner menu (397 calories)
*½ baked Oriental chicken breast (154 calories)
*½ baked acorn squash (70 calories)
½ cucumber, peeled and sliced (10 calories) and 1 scallion, finely chopped
    (4 calories); toss with 2 tablespoons white vinegar and serve on 3 Boston
    lettuce leaves, torn into bite-sized pieces (3 calories)
1 breadstick (40 calories)
1 orange, peeled and sliced (64 calories), with 2 tablespoons vanilla yogurt
    (25 calories) and 1 tablespoon toasted wheat germ (27 calories)
Coffee (regular or decafeinated) or tea (no sugar or milk)

*Baked Oriental chicken breast

1 12-ounce chicken breast, cut in half (288 calories)
1 tablespoon soy sauce (10 calories)
1 tablespoon lemon juice (3 calories)
1 clove garlic, minced (3 calories)
1 slice fresh ginger, grated, or ¼ teaspoon ground ginger
1 scallion, finely sliced (4 calories)

Place chicken in small bowl. Combine soy sauce, lemon juice, garlic, ginger, and scallion; pour over chicken. Marinate chicken for 1 hour or more, turning several times to make sure pieces are well coated with marinade. Remove chicken from marinade and place in shallow baking pan. Bake in a 350° oven for 45 to 55 minutes until done. Save ½ chicken breast for lunch on Day 8.

*Baked acorn squash

1 12-ounce acorn squash, cut in half and cleaned (108 calories)
1 teaspoon margarine (33 calories)
¼ teaspoon cinnamon

Place squash, cut side down, in small baking pan into which you have put ½ inch water. Cook in a 350° oven for 30 minutes; then turn cut side up and brush with softened margarine. Sprinkle with cinnamon and continue cooking for another 15 minutes or until done. Save ½ for dinner on Day 8.

Eleven o'clock exercise break: mat exercises to relax you and tone your muscles.

Pelvic twist

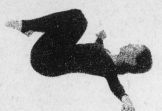

1. Lie on your back, arms out at shoulder level. Inhaling, raise both knees and bring as close to body as possible.

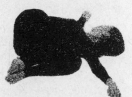

2. Exhaling, roll to the right so that right knee and ankle touch floor. Roll over to the left, touching floor. Roll to each side 5 times.

Reverse leg lifts

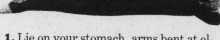

1. Lie on your stomach, arms bent at elbows and chin resting on hands.

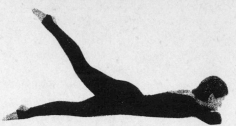

2. Keeping it straight, lift right leg straight up as high as possible. Hold for a count of 5.

3. Repeat with left leg. Alternate, lifting each leg 5 times.

Last thing before you go to bed: **relaxation technique.** Read exercise all the way through before you do it.

Lie on your back on a mat, with legs slightly separated and relaxed, arms at your sides, palms of hands facing up. Lift your right leg and shake it vigorously. Let it drop to the mat. Do the same with your left leg. Then shake your right arm and let it drop to the mat. Do the same with your left arm. Lie quietly, breathing in and out deeply 3 times. Lift your hands and clasp your neck. Massage the back of your neck gently and thoroughly and then massage behind your ears. Return arms to sides and inhale deeply 3 times.

Monday

Morning

On arising: **breathing exercise.** Sit very tall on the edge of the bed with feet planted firmly on the floor. Rest hands on thighs, palms up. Keep your eyes closed throughout this exercise.

Exhale completely. Inhale by taking a series of short breaths until lungs are completely full. Pause for a moment. Now exhale slowly and thoroughly, making a *hahhh* sound as you do so. Inhale again, in a series of short breaths, and repeat entire exercise for 3 minutes.

Immediately after breathing exercise: **wake-up exercises.**

Side stretch

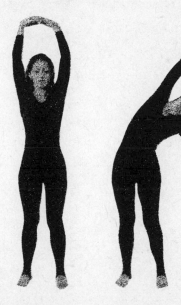

1. Stand with feet 6 inches apart. Breathe in deeply as you lift arms above head, placing one hand over the other.

2. Exhaling, bend to the left as far as is comfortable.

3. Go back to the center, breathing in. As you exhale, bend to the right as far as is comfortable. Stretch 10 times to each side.

Running in place. Always run on a carpeted or padded surface. Warm up with a slow jog of 40 steps. Rest for a moment and then run at a faster pace for 2 minutes. Cool down by walking around, taking long strides, until your pulse rate and breathing have returned to normal.

Weigh yourself and record your weight.

Breakfast menu (234 calories)
1 4-ounce glass orange juice (55 calories)
¼ cup pineapple cottage cheese, to use as spread on toast (70 calories)
1 slice cracked wheat toast (65 calories)
1 4-ounce glass skim milk (44 calories)
Coffee (regular or decaffeinated) or tea (no sugar)

Brown-bag lunch: If you are taking lunch to your office, prepare it right after breakfast.

"It is praiseworthy even to attempt a great action."
— LA ROCHEFOUCAULD

Monday

Daytime

Midmorning break: **herb tea.**

Lunch menu (255 calories)
*Chef's salad with slivered chicken (191 calories)
3 melba toast rounds (24 calories)
½ banana (40 calories)
Coffee (regular or decaffeinated) or tea (no sugar or milk)

*Chef's salad with slivered chicken

3 ounces chicken, slivered (use ½ baked Oriental chicken breast reserved from Day 7) (154 calories)

4 leaves romaine lettuce, torn into small pieces (10 calories)

½ cucumber, peeled and cubed (10 calories)

2 scallions, thinly sliced (8 calories)

1 tablespoon parsley, chopped (2 calories)

1 tablespoon low-calorie Italian salad dressing (7 calories)

Combine all the ingredients and toss. Add salad dressing just before serving and toss to coat the ingredients.

Midafternoon break: **breathing and stretching.** Do 3 minutes of the short-breath breathing you did this morning. Stretch and move around. Walk to a colleague's office or to another part of the house. Get your circulation going. Relax after cooling off with a 4-ounce glass of tomato juice (23 calories).

8 | Monday

Evening

Dinner menu (456 calories)

*Vealburger with lemon and marjoram (202 calories)
2 stalks broccoli, steamed (36 calories) and sprinkled with 1
   teaspoon lemon juice (1 calorie)
½ acorn squash (reheated from Day 7) (70 calories)
2 breadsticks (80 calories)
½ banana, sliced (40 calories) in 2 ounces fresh orange juice (27 calories)
Coffee (regular or decaffeinated) or tea (no sugar or milk)

*Vealburger with lemon and marjoram

¼ pound ground veal (196 calories)
1 tablespoon onion, finely chopped
   (5 calories)
¼ teaspoon grated lemon rind

1 teaspoon lemon juice (1 calorie)
¼ teaspoon marjoram
¼ teaspoon salt
⅛ teaspoon freshly ground black pepper

Combine all ingredients and mix thoroughly. Shape veal into patty. Flatten it to about ½ inch. Broil 4 inches from flame for 5 minutes per side.

Eleven o'clock exercise break: mat exercises to relax you and tone your muscles.

Reverse leg lifts

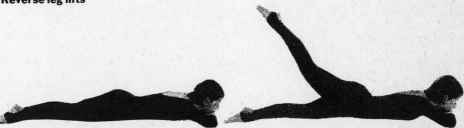

1. Lie on your stomach, arms bent at elbows and chin resting on hands.

2. Keeping it straight, lift right leg straight up as high as possible. Hold for a count of 5.

3. Repeat with left leg. Alternate, lifting each leg 5 times.

Knee and head lifts

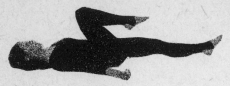 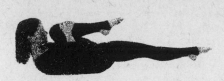

1. Lie on your back, arms at sides, palms down. Bend right knee and pull toward chest.

2. Inhaling, grasp leg with hands just below knee. At the same time, raise head and touch forehead to knee. Exhaling, return to starting position. Repeat 10 times.

Last thing before you go to bed: **nature meditation.** Read through before starting.

Lie on your back on a mat, with your legs slightly separated and relaxed and your arms at your sides, palms of hands facing up. Imagine you are walking on a country road. It is spring, and the apple orchards are in bloom. You cross over a stile fence and walk among the blossoming trees. It is early morning, and the trees smell fragrant and rich. The flowers are white, edged in pale pink, and there are thousands of them. Birds fly from tree to tree. Sit down under one of the trees and absorb the beauty around you.

Tuesday

Morning

On arising: **breathing exercise.** Sit very tall on the edge of your bed with your feet planted firmly on the floor. Rest hands on thighs, palms up. Keep your eyes closed throughout this exercise. Exhale completely. Inhale by taking a series of short breaths until lungs are completely full. Pause for a moment.

Now, exhale slowly and thoroughly, making a *hahhh* sound as you do so. Repeat for a 3-minute period.

Immediately after breathing exercise: **wake-up exercises.**

Alternate arm stretch

1. Stand with feet together. Breathe in deeply as you lift right arm straight up. Now, stretch right arm up and left arm down. Hold for a few seconds.

2. Drop right arm and relax. Repeat, lifting and stretching left arm up and right arm down. Hold for a few seconds, then drop left arm and relax. Alternate arms 10 times.

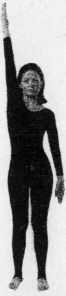

Running in place. Always run on a carpeted or padded surface. Warm up with a slow jog for 40 steps. After you have warmed up, rest for a moment and then run at a faster pace. Run for 2 minutes. Cool down by walking around, taking long strides, until your pulse rate and breathing have returned to normal.

Weigh yourself and record your weight.

Breakfast menu (240 calories)

1 4-ounce glass orange juice (55 calories)
¾ cup bran flakes (101 calories)
½ banana, sliced (40 calories)
1 4-ounce glass skim milk (44 calories)
Coffee (regular or decaffeinated) or tea (no sugar)

Brown-bag lunch: If you are taking lunch to your office, prepare it immediately after breakfast.

Tuesday

Daytime

Midmorning break: **herb tea.**

Lunch menu (252 calories)
*Spinach salad with hard-cooked egg (188 calories)
3 melba toast rounds (24 calories)
½ banana (40 calories)
Coffee (regular or decaffeinated) or tea (no sugar or milk)

*Spinach salad with hard-cooked egg

½ pound fresh spinach, washed, dried, and stems removed (44 calories)
1 hard-cooked egg, chopped (78 calories)
4 mushrooms, sliced (32 calories)

4 cherry tomatoes, halved (16 calories)
1 scallion, finely sliced (4 calories)
2 tablespoons low-calorie Italian salad dressing (14 calories)

Hard-cook egg by putting it into cold water and bringing to a boil. Lower heat and simmer for 6 minutes. Turn off heat and let egg stand for 15 minutes. Tear spinach leaves into bite-sized pieces. Combine all ingredients and toss thoroughly. If you prepare salad in the morning, do not add dressing until just before eating.

Midafternoon break: Run in place for one minute. After cooling off, have a cup of herb tea.

Tuesday

Evening

Dinner menu (502 calories)

¼ pound cooked ham steak, grilled in nonstick frying pan (213 calories)

½ cup green peas, steamed (68 calories), mixed with 1 sliced scallion (4 calories)

Tossed green salad made from 2 cups romaine and Boston lettuce leaves, torn into bite-sized pieces (15 calories) and 1 tablespoon chopped parsley (2 calories); serve with 1 tablespoon lemon-cumin salad dressing (50 calories)

1 slice cracked wheat bread (65 calories)

⅓ cup coffee yogurt (67 calories), sprinkled with 1 tablespoon roasted, slivered almonds (18 calories)

Beauty break: **applying lipstick with a brush.** Lipstick looks better and lasts longer when you apply it with a brush. And you use less lipstick to achieve the look you want. Learning to use a brush like a professional takes practice, but it isn't hard to master. Try combining colors to get just the look you want.

You will need: a good-quality lipstick brush, plum or rosy-brown lipstick, pink-beige lipstick, pot of clear gloss (optional), and hand-held magnifying mirror.

Outline your mouth with the darker shade of lipstick and fill in with the lighter one. To outline, dip the brush in the plum or rosy-brown lipstick. Beginning in the center of the upper lip, draw a line at the edge of the lip. Steady your hand by resting the little finger on your chin. Outline bottom lip by starting at the corner and brushing toward the center. Next, fill in with the lighter color. If you like the shiny effect that gloss gives, use the brush to cover your mouth with gloss. Make-up experts are unanimous in advising against trying to change the shape of your mouth. Models can do this for photographs, but it is not attractive in everyday life.

Eleven o'clock exercise break: mat exercises to relax you and tone your muscles.

Leg up and over

Knee bends and squeeze

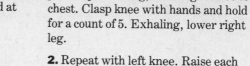

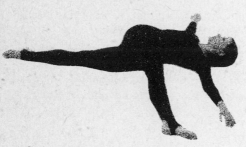

1. Lie on your back, arms extended at shoulder level. Bend right knee.

1. Lie on your back, arms at sides and palms up. Inhaling, raise right knee to chest. Clasp knee with hands and hold for a count of 5. Exhaling, lower right leg.

2. Repeat with left knee. Raise each knee 5 times.

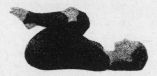

2. Straighten leg up into air, toes pointed. Hold for a count of 3.

3. Raise both knees together. Clasp with hands and pull in for a count of 5. Straighten legs and lower slowly. Repeat 5 times with both legs.

3. Swing leg over to touch floor on left side as close to left hand as possible. Keep arms and head stationary. Swing leg back to center and lower. Repeat with left leg. Do each leg 5 times.

Morning

On arising: **breathing exercise.** Sit very tall on the edge of the bed with feet planted firmly on the floor. Rest hands on thighs, palms facing up. Keep your eyes closed throughout this exercise.

Exhale completely. Inhale by taking a series of short breaths until lungs are completely full. Pause for a moment. Now exhale slowly and thoroughly, making a *hahhh* sound as you do so. Inhale again, taking short breaths, and repeat entire exercise. Do this breathing exercise for 3 minutes.

Immediately after breathing exercise: **wake-up exercises.**

Arm and leg stretch

1. Stand with feet together, arms down at sides. Stretch right arm up and forward and left leg back, pointing toes. Stretch fully without straining. Hold position for a count of 5.

2. Repeat, lifting left arm up and extending right leg back. Alternate 10 times to a side.

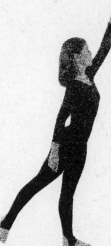

Running in place. Always run on a carpeted or padded surface. Warm up with a slow jog of 40 steps. Rest for a moment and then run at a faster pace for 2 minutes. Cool down by walking around, taking long strides, until your pulse rate and breathing have returned to normal.

Weigh yourself and record your weight.

Breakfast menu (235 calories)
½ grapefruit (48 calories)
1 egg, soft-cooked (78 calories)
1 slice cracked wheat toast (65 calories)
1 4-ounce glass skim milk (44 calories)
Coffee (regular or decaffeinated) or tea (no sugar)

Brown-bag lunch: If you are taking lunch to your office, prepare it right after breakfast.

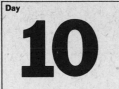

10 | Wednesday

Daytime

Midmorning break: **herb tea.**

Lunch menu (276 calories)
*Tuna salad with capers (202 calories)
3 melba toast rounds (24 calories)
½ cup green grapes (50 calories)
Coffee (regular or decaffeinated) or tea (no sugar or milk)

*Tuna salad with capers
1 3½-ounce can solid white tuna,
  water-packed (120 calories)
1 teaspoon capers (3 calories)
1 scallion, thinly sliced (4 calories)
½ cucumber, peeled and chopped
  (10 calories)

2 cups Boston lettuce, torn into
  bite-sized pieces (15 calories)
1 tablespoon lemon-cumin salad dressing
  (50 calories)

Combine tuna, capers, scallion, and cucumber. Toss to mix thoroughly. Serve on bed of lettuce. Drizzle dressing over all immediately before serving.

Midafternoon break: Stretch and do 5 deep inhalations and exhalations. Run in place for a minute. After cooling off, drink a cup of herb tea.

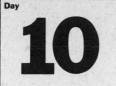

Wednesday

Evening

Dinner menu (464 calories)
1 11-ounce glass mineral water with ice and a thin slice of lemon
*Shrimp marinara (164 calories)
2 stalks broccoli, steamed (36 calories)
½ cup cooked white rice (112 calories)
*Baked banana with brown sugar and orange juice (108 calories)
Cappuccino (made with ½ cup instant espresso and ½ cup hot skim milk,
   sprinkled with cinnamon) (44 calories)

*Shrimp marinara

10 raw shrimp
  (100 calories)
½ can (4 ounces) tomato sauce
  (40 calories)
½ onion, chopped (19 calories)
1 clove garlic, minced (3 calories)

¼ teaspoon oregano
¼ teaspoon basil
¼ cup water
1 tablespoon parsley, chopped
  (2 calories)

If shrimp are fresh, clean and devein. Plunge them into lightly salted boiling water for 3 minutes. If frozen, follow package directions for cooking. Combine tomato sauce, garlic, onion, and herbs and simmer for about 20 minutes. As sauce thickens, gradually add the water. Add shrimp and simmer for several minutes until shrimp are heated through. Sprinkle with chopped fresh parsley.

*Baked banana with brown sugar and orange juice

1 banana, peeled and cut in two
  lengthwise (80 calories)

2 tablespoons orange juice (14 calories)
1 teaspoon brown sugar (14 calories)

Place banana, cut side down, in small baking dish. Sprinkle with orange juice and then with sugar. Bake in a 350° oven until done, about 30 minutes.

Eleven o'clock exercise break: mat exercises to relax you and tone your muscles.

Pelvic lift

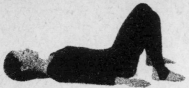

1. Lie on your back, arms at sides and palms down. Bend knees and place feet flat on floor, as close to buttocks as possible.

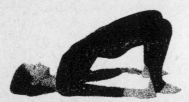

2. Inhaling, raise buttocks and arch back. Hold for a count of 5. Exhaling, return to starting position. Repeat 10 times.

Pelvic twist with extended legs

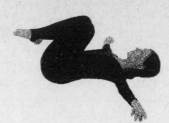

1. Lie on your back, arms out at shoulder level. Inhaling, raise both knees and bring as close to body as possible.

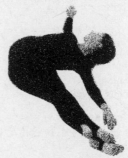

2. Roll to the right, straightening legs. Lower legs to floor. Bring legs back to center bent position. Repeat, rolling to the left. Roll to each side 3 times.

Last thing before you go to bed: **relaxation technique.** Read through the exercise before you start.

Lie flat on your back on the mat. Legs should be relaxed. Arms are close to your sides, palms of hands facing up. Close your eyes and take two deep breaths. With your mind's eye, you are going to touch each part of your body and relax it. Start with your toes. Imagine you can touch your big toe with your mind; relax it. Move from toe to toe on the right foot. Then, as though your mind had a kind of relaxing ray, move up to the right ankle, the shin, the knee, the thigh. Now do your left foot and leg. Slowly cover the entire body, including the top of the head, the ears, the back of the head, the nape of the neck, and the spine, always focusing the beam of your mind on each part of your body to relax it. When you have finished, lie quietly for a few minutes and concentrate on your deep breathing.

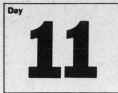

11 | Thursday

Morning

On arising: **breathing exercise.** Sit very tall on the edge of the bed with feet planted firmly on the floor. Rest hands on thighs, palms facing up. Keep your eyes closed throughout this exercise.

Exhale completely. Inhale by taking a series of short breaths until lungs are completely full. Pause for a moment. Now exhale slowly and thoroughly, making a *hahhh* sound as you do so. Inhale again, in a series of short breaths. Repeat entire exercise several times for a 3-minute period.

Immediately after breathing exercise: **wake-up exercises.**

Fencer's lunge

1. Stand with feet 2½ feet apart. Raise arms to shoulder height. Bend right knee and shift weight to the right. Hold for a count of 5 and return to center.

2. Bend left knee and shift weight to the left. Hold for a count of 5 and return to center. Repeat 10 times to each side.

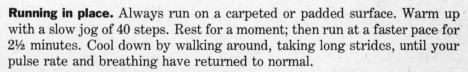

Running in place. Always run on a carpeted or padded surface. Warm up with a slow jog of 40 steps. Rest for a moment; then run at a faster pace for 2½ minutes. Cool down by walking around, taking long strides, until your pulse rate and breathing have returned to normal.

Weigh yourself and record your weight.

Breakfast menu (233 calories)
½ grapefruit (48 calories)
¾ cup bran flakes (101 calories)
1 4-ounce glass skim milk (44 calories)
½ cup blueberries (fresh or unsweetened frozen) (40 calories)
Coffee (regular or decaffeinated) or tea (no sugar)

Brown-bag lunch: If you are taking lunch to your office, prepare it immediately after breakfast.

Note: Transfer flank steak from freezer to refrigerator.

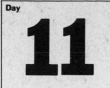

Thursday

Daytime

Midmorning break: **herb tea.**

Lunch menu (313 calories)
*Fruit and cottage cheese salad (273 calories)
1 breadstick (40 calories)
Coffee (regular or decaffeinated) or tea (no sugar or milk)

*Fruit and cottage cheese salad

½ cup cottage cheese (120 calories)
½ cup strawberries (26 calories)
½ apple, cored and cut in cubes
   (45 calories)
¼ cup vanilla yogurt (50 calories)

1 tablespoon toasted wheat germ
   (27 calories)
2 leaves romaine lettuce, torn into
   bite-sized pieces (5 calories)

Place cottage cheese on bed of lettuce. Cover with fruit and then with yogurt. Sprinkle wheat germ over all.

Midafternoon break: Run in place for 1 minute. After cooling off, drink a cup of herb tea.

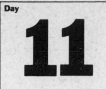
Evening

Dinner menu (511 calories)

*Broiled marinated flank steak (232 calories)

Baked potato (Wash potato, prick with fork, and bake for 45 minutes to 1 hour in 400° oven until soft.) (90 calories)

*Baked herb-seasoned tomato (47 calories)

Tossed green salad made from 2 cups romaine and Boston lettuce leaves, torn into bite-sized pieces (15 calories) and 1 tablespoon chopped parsley (2 calories); serve with 1 tablespoon low-calorie Italian salad dressing (7 calories).

½ cup coffee yogurt (100 calories), sprinkled with 1 tablespoon roasted, slivered almonds (18 calories)

Coffee (regular or decaffeinated) or tea (no sugar or milk)

*Broiled marinated flank steak

¼ pound flank steak (224 calories)
1 tablespoon soy sauce (10 calories)
1 clove garlic, minced (3 calories)

1 tablespoon lemon juice (3 calories)
¼ teaspoon onion powder

Put flank steak in a glass bowl or dish. Combine soy sauce, lemon juice, garlic, and onion. Pour over flank steak. Marinate for an hour or more. Remove steak from marinade and put under preheated broiler, 4 inches from flame. Broil for 5 minutes on each side or until done to your taste. Slice steak in thin diagonal slices with a sharp knife.

*Baked herb-seasoned tomato

1 tomato (44 calories)
1 clove garlic, minced (3 calories)

Pinch of oregano
Black pepper, freshly ground

Wash tomato and remove stem end. Cut in half and place in small baking dish. Sprinkle garlic, oregano, and black pepper to taste over tops of tomatoes. Bake in 400° oven for 10 to 15 minutes.

Beauty break: **give yourself a professional manicure.** For beautiful nails, make a once-a-week manicure part of your beauty program. When you allow adequate time for this program and use the proper equipment, you will discover that it is a relaxing and sensuous experience.

You will need: a small bowl of warm soapy water, 2 cotton pads, 1 emery board, cuticle remover, nail clippers, orangewood stick, nail polish and polish remover, and finish coat.

If you are wearing polish, remove it with a cotton pad moistened with a conditioning polish remover. Shake hands vigorously for several minutes to relax tension. With an emery board, file nails in one direction only. Do not file into the corners of the nail. Leave sides straight to prevent splitting.

File tips of nails into a slightly curved, squared-off shape. Wash hands in warm water with a mild soap. Next, soak nails for several minutes in bowl of warm water and a mild detergent.

When cuticles are soft, apply cuticle remover very gently with orangewood stick wrapped in wisps of cotton from one of the cotton pads. After 3 minutes, gently push back cuticle with the cotton-wrapped orangewood stick. Trim any hangnails with the clipper, but do not cut the cuticle itself. Soak nails again in soapy water. Dry thoroughly. (Drying is especially important if you are using polish. Polish applied to dry, oil-free nails lasts longer.) If you do not wear polish, you might like to try nail buffing, which achieves a natural yet finished look. There are several good nail-buffing kits available at your local pharmacy.

Some nail-care do's and don'ts

Do wear gloves for dishwashing, household chores, and gardening.

Do use a nail-conditioning cream or a hand cream at bedtime, especially in winter.

Do establish nail upkeep as a part of your weekly beauty program.

Do let polish dry for several hours before putting your hands in water.

Don't use your nails to open stubborn boxes or as tools to fix things.

Don't have nails at different lengths or exotically long. Hands with some short and some long nails are unattractive. If a nail breaks off, file other nails to give your hands balance or repair nails with a repair kit.

Eleven o'clock exercise break: mat exercises to relax you and tone your muscles.

Seated leg extension

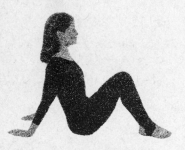 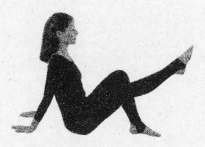

1. Sit with hands placed behind you and knees bent.

2. Extend right leg straight up and then lower.

3. Repeat with left leg. Alternate, lifting each leg 3 times.

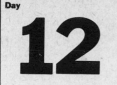

Friday

Morning

On arising: **breathing exercise.** Sit very tall on the edge of the bed with feet planted firmly on the floor. Rest hands on thighs, palms facing up. Keep your eyes closed throughout this exercise.

Exhale completely. Inhale by taking a series of short breaths until lungs are completely full. Pause for a moment. Now exhale slowly and thoroughly, making a *hahhh* sound as you do so. Inhale, again taking short breaths, and repeat entire exercise for a 3-minute period.

Immediately after breathing exercise: **wake-up exercises.**

Clasped hand stretch

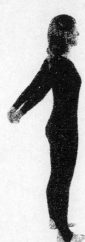
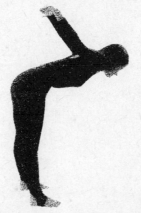

1. Stand with feet 3 inches apart. Link fingers behind back.

2. Lean forward from the hips and lift arms.

3. Lean as far forward as comfortable. Straighten up and return to starting position. Repeat 10 times.

Running in place. Always run on a carpeted or padded surface. Warm up with a slow jog of 40 steps. Rest for a moment, then run at a faster pace for 2½ minutes. Cool down by walking around, taking long strides, until your pulse rate and breathing have returned to normal.

Weigh yourself and record your weight.

Breakfast menu (224 calories)
1 4-ounce glass orange juice (55 calories)
1 slice cracked wheat toast (65 calories)
¼ cup cottage cheese, sprinkled with cinnamon, to use as spread on toast (60 calories)
1 4-ounce glass skim milk (44 calories)
Coffee (regular or decaffeinated) or tea (no sugar)

Brown-bag lunch: If you are taking lunch to your office, prepare it immediately after breakfast.

Note: Transfer chicken breast from freezer to refrigerator.

"Self-trust is the first secret of success."
—EMERSON

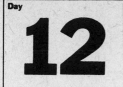

Friday

Daytime

Midmorning break: **herb tea.**

Lunch menu (264 calories)
*Open-faced tuna salad sandwich (224 calories)
½ apple (40 calories)
Coffee (regular or decaffeinated) or tea (no sugar or milk)

*Open-faced tuna salad sandwich

1 3½-ounce can solid white tuna, water-packed (120 calories)
1 teaspoon capers (3 calories)
1 tablespoon parsley, chopped (2 calories)

2 teaspoons imitation or diet mayonnaise (32 calories)
1 leaf romaine lettuce (2 calories)
1 slice cracked wheat bread (65 calories)

Combine drained tuna, capers, chopped parsley, and mayonnaise and mix thoroughly. Tear romaine lettuce leaf into small pieces. Cover bread with lettuce, then with the tuna salad.

Midafternoon break: Run in place for 1 minute. After cooling off, have a cup of herb tea.

Prevention's Ultimate Diet
recipes

Chicken-Cranberry Sandwich

PREP TIME **5 minutes**

Smear 2 tablespoons softened reduced-fat cream cheese onto 1 slice whole grain bread (toasted or untoasted). Spread 2 tablespoons cranberry chutney, sauce, or relish onto another toasted slice. Fill sandwich with thinly sliced reduced-fat Cheddar cheese (about 1 ounce), thinly sliced chicken breast (about 2 ounces), apple slices, and a handful of trimmed watercress or baby spinach leaves.

Makes 1 sandwich

PER SERVING 398 cal, 33 g pro, 40 g carb, 13 g fat, 7 g sat fat, 85 mg chol, 12 g fiber, 449 mg sodium

% CAL 32% pro, 39% carb, 29% fat

Soup for All Seasons

(see "More Seasonal Soup Suggestions," next page, for year-round options)

PREP TIME **15 minutes**

COOKING TIME **35 minutes**

- 1 Tbsp canola oil
- 1 tsp butter
- 1 med onion, sliced
- 2 bay leaves
- 1 lg butternut squash, peeled, seeded, and thinly sliced
- 3 ripe pears, peeled and chopped
- 1/3 tsp garam masala spice mixture*
- 1/4 tsp ground red pepper
- 5 c reduced-sodium vegetable or chicken broth
- 1 med potato, peeled and cut into 1" cubes
- 1/2 tsp salt
- 1/3 c whole milk
  - Low-fat plain yogurt (garnish)
  - Fresh herbs (garnish)

*Available at specialty grocery stores or *www.ethnicgrocer.com*

1. In large saucepan, heat oil and butter over medium heat. Add onion and bay leaves and cook, stirring often, until softened, about 5 minutes. Increase heat to medium-high, add squash, pears, garam masala, and pepper, and cook, stirring occasionally, 5 minutes longer or until squash and pears begin to brown.

2. Add broth, potato, and salt. Bring mixture to a boil, reduce heat, and simmer until squash is very soft, about 20 to 25 minutes. Remove bay leaves.

3. Puree soup in batches in food processor or blender. Return to saucepan, stir in milk, and bring to a simmer. Divide into 6 bowls, garnish and serve.

Makes 6 (1/2-cup) servings

PER SERVING 215 cal, 9 g pro, 34 g carb, 6 g fat, 1.5 g sat fat, 27 mg chol, 3 g fiber, 420 mg sodium

% CAL 15% pro, 60% carb, 25% fat

DIET FREEDOM!

Freedom from hunger, from counting, and from yo-yo dieting!

Lose weight and eat great **FREE for an entire week**, with NutriSystem® Nourish™!

Freedom from hunger!

Choose from **100 deliciously prepared, perfectly portioned foods,** including favorites like hearty lasagna and tasty chocolates. Plus, the NEW NutriSystem Nourish food program is low in fat and rich in "good carbs," so **you'll burn more fat** while eating the foods you love!

Freedom from counting carbs, calories or points!

With NutriSystem, you don't have to count carbs, calories or anything else. You simply eat delicious food, plus **everything is delivered right to your door, ready to heat, eat and go!** And all for less than $10 a day!

Freedom from yo-yo dieting!

Now you can eat healthier, five times a day! NutriSystem is the program that will empower you to break free from the ups and downs of fad diets.

after

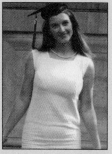

"I ate chocolate and lost 20 lbs."

before

"What I really love is the convenience. I don't have to plan, measure or weigh anything... **not to mention I get to eat chips and chocolate!"**

–Television's **Zora Andrich**

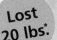

Lost 20 lbs.*

*Results not typical

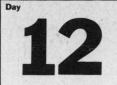
Friday

Evening

Relaxation technique: **lying on a slant board.** A good revitalizer for the end of the day is to lie for 10 to 15 minutes on a slant board. Cover eyes with cotton pads soaked in tea or witch hazel. If you don't have a slant board, simply lie on your bed with legs elevated against the wall or lie on a mat on the floor with legs resting on a low stool.

Dinner menu (540 calories)
1 11-ounce glass mineral water with ice and a thin slice of lemon
*Chinese chicken with curry flavor (205 calories)
½ cup cooked white rice (112 calories)
2 medium stalks broccoli, steamed (36 calories)
Tossed green salad made from 2 cups Boston and romaine lettuce leaves, torn into bite-sized pieces (15 calories) and 1 carrot, grated (17 calories); serve with 1 tablespoon low-calorie Italian salad dressing (7 calories) (50 calories).
1 orange, peeled and sliced (64 calories) and ¼ cup blueberries (20 calories) in 2 tablespoons orange juice (14 calories)
Coffee (regular or decaffeinated) or tea (no sugar or milk)

*Chinese chicken with curry flavor
1 12-ounce chicken breast, cut in half (288 calories)
1 teaspoon safflower oil (40 calories)
1 onion, sliced (38 calories)
1 teaspoon curry powder
½ can (4 ounces) tomato sauce (40 calories)
½ cup chicken stock, made from bouillon cube (3 calories)

Put safflower oil in nonstick pan. Add sliced onion and sauté onions for a few minutes. Don't brown onions, just soften. Add curry powder and stir to blend well. Cook over medium heat for 1 or 2 minutes. Add chicken and cook quickly to brown slightly. Add tomato sauce and chicken stock and bring to a boil. Lower heat and simmer for about 40 minutes, covered. Add more stock if necessary. Remove chicken from sauce when cooked and serve ½ of the breast and sauce. Use ½ for lunch on Day 13.

Eleven o'clock exercise break: mat exercises to relax you and tone your muscles

Roll ups

Seated body stretch

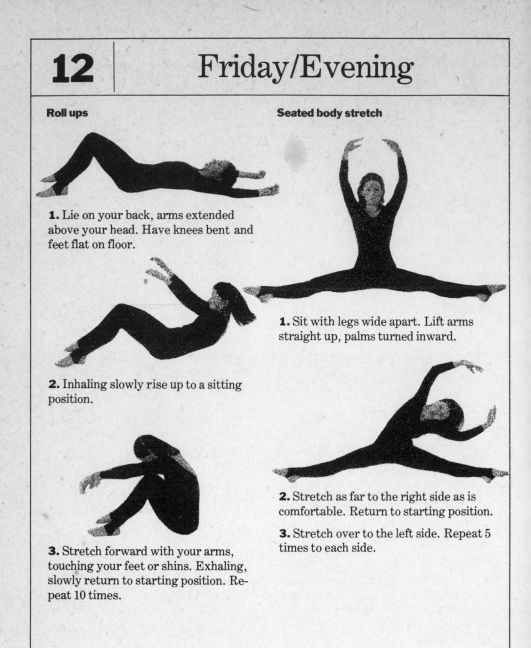

1. Lie on your back, arms extended above your head. Have knees bent and feet flat on floor.

2. Inhaling slowly rise up to a sitting position.

3. Stretch forward with your arms, touching your feet or shins. Exhaling, slowly return to starting position. Repeat 10 times.

1. Sit with legs wide apart. Lift arms straight up, palms turned inward.

2. Stretch as far to the right side as is comfortable. Return to starting position.

3. Stretch over to the left side. Repeat 5 times to each side.

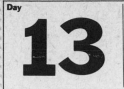 13 | Saturday

---

Morning

On arising: **breathing exercise.** Sit very tall on the edge of the bed with feet planted firmly on the floor. Rest hands on thighs, palms facing up. Keep your eyes closed throughout this exercise.

Exhale completely. Inhale by taking a series of short breaths until lungs are completely full. Pause for a moment. Now exhale slowly and thoroughly, making a *hahhh* sound as you do so. Inhale again, taking short breaths, and repeat entire exercise several times for a 3-minute period.

Immediately after breathing exercise: **wake-up exercises.**

Alternate arm stretch

1. Stand with feet together. Breathe in deeply as you lift right arm straight up. Now, stretch right arm up and left arm down. Hold for a few seconds.

2. Drop right arm and relax. Repeat, lifting and stretching left arm up and right arm down. Hold for a few seconds, then drop left arm and relax. Alternate arms 10 times.

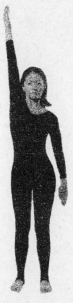

Running in place. Always run on a carpeted or padded surface. Warm up with a slow jog of 40 steps. Rest for a moment, then run at a faster pace for 2½ minutes. Cool down by walking around, taking long strides, until your pulse rate and breathing have returned to normal.

Weigh yourself and record your weight.

Breakfast menu (213 calories)
1 egg, scrambled in nonstick pan (78 calories) with 1 tablespoon grated
    Swiss cheese (26 calories)
1 slice cracked wheat toast (65 calories)
1 4-ounce glass skim milk (44 calories)
Coffee (regular or decaffeinated) or tea (no sugar)

Shopping List

Breads

1 loaf whole wheat bread (18 slices)

Dairy products

1 8-ounce container cottage cheese
2 quarts skim milk
1 8-ounce container coffee yogurt
1 8-ounce container vanilla yogurt

Fruits and vegetables

1 3-inch apple
1 7-inch banana
4 3-inch oranges
4 lemons
2 2½-inch tangerines
1 4-inch grapefruit
1 3-inch pear
1 8-ounce can pineapple chunks, in own
juice
2 heads Boston lettuce
1 head celery
2 7-inch cucumbers
¼ pound medium mushrooms (about 8)
1 pound onions (4 to a pound)
1 bunch parsley
2 heads romaine lettuce
½ pound small new potatoes (6 to a
pound)
1 baking potato (about ¼ pound)
1 pound regular potatoes (3 to a pound)
1 bunch scallions
1 1-pint carton cherry tomatoes
2 8¼-ounce cans whole tomatoes
1 6-inch zucchini

Meat and fish

¼ pound steak, cut into 1″ cubes
1 12-ounce chicken breast
1 6-ounce boneless chicken breast (store
in freezer)
½ pound ground beef round
1 4-ounce center-cut pork chop (store in
freezer)
¼ pound veal for scaloppine (store in
freezer)
2 3½-ounce cans solid white tuna,
water-packed

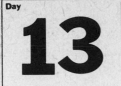

Daytime

Lunch menu (275 calories)

Chinese chicken with curry flavor (Reheat ½ breast in sauce and serve with remaining sauce.) (204 calories)

Tossed green salad made from ¼ head iceberg lettuce, shredded (10 calories); serve with 1 tablespoon low-calorie bleu-cheese salad dressing (12 calories)

3 melba toast rounds (24 calories)

¼ cup green grapes (25 calories)

Coffee (regular or decaffeinated) or tea (no sugar or milk)

Beauty break: **applying makeup for the natural look.** Many makeup experts recommend using a small sponge to apply foundation and blusher. This simple yet effective technique helps to achieve that desired soft, natural look, and it avoids streaking and lines of demarcation. Also, makeup applied this way tends to last longer.

You will need: mild soap, moisturizer, 2 small makeup sponges (foam rubber or natural), toning lotion or water to dampen sponges, lightweight foundation, and powder or cream blusher.

Wash face and neck with mild soap and warm water. Rinse thoroughly and pat dry. Apply a light layer of moisturizer (don't forget your neck). Wet the sponge and squeeze almost dry. Apply a small amount of foundation and smooth on. When you have applied foundation to your face and neck, you are ready to apply blusher. Use a different sponge for this. Dampen the sponge and this time use a small amount of blusher. Apply on the "apple" of the cheeks, where color would normally be, not high on the cheekbones and temples.

Beauty break checklist for upcoming week

Alcohol or witch hazel

Cotton pads

Old toothbrush

Eyebrow tweezers

Medicated moisture lotion

Magnifying mirror

Eye shadow

Eyeliner

Eyelash curler

Mascara

13 | Saturday

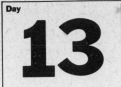

Evening

Dinner menu (490 calories)
1 11-ounce glass mineral water with ice and a thin slice lemon
*Shish kebab (307 calories)
½ cup cooked white rice (112 calories)
Tossed green salad made from 2 cups romaine and Boston lettuce leaves,
 torn into bite-sized pieces (15 calories) and ½ cucumber, peeled and sliced
 (10 calories); serve with 1 tablespoon low-calorie Italian salad dressing
 (7 calories)
1 tangerine (39 calories)
Coffee (regular or decaffeinated) or tea (no sugar or milk)

*Shish kebab
¼ pound round steak, cut into 1-inch
 cubes (224 calories)
4 cherry tomatoes (16 calories)
1 green pepper, seeded and cut
 into squares (16 calories)
2 mushrooms (10 calories)

1 onion, cut into half (38 calories)
2 tablespoons lemon juice (6 calories)
¼ teaspoon thyme
¼ teaspoon salt
Pinch of pepper

Combine lemon juice, thyme, salt, and pepper in a mixing bowl. Add meat cubes and
thoroughly coat with marinade. Refrigerate meat for 3 to 4 hours. To broil, thread
meat on skewers, alternating cubes with tomatoes, green peppers, onions, and
mushrooms. Broil about 4 inches from flame, basting with marinade and turning
skewers to brown evenly. Broil for about 10 minutes.

Eleven o'clock exercise break: mat exercises to relax you and tone your
muscles.

Pelvic lift

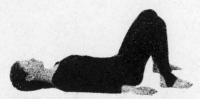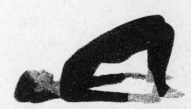

1. Lie on your back, arms at sides and
palms down. Bend knees and place feet
flat on floor, as close to buttocks as possible.

2. Inhaling, raise buttocks and arch
back. Hold for a count of 5. Exhaling, return to starting position. Repeat 10
times.

Seated leg extension

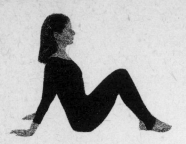 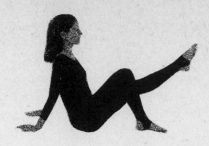

1. Sit with hands placed behind you and knees bent.

2. Extend right leg straight up and then lower.

3. Repeat with left leg. Alternate, lifting each leg 3 times.

Morning

On arising: **breathing exercise.** Stand by the side of your bed with your spine straight and your feet firmly placed a few inches apart. As you breathe in, lift up your rib cage. Keep your eyes closed while you do the exercise. Concentrate totally on your breathing.

Begin by exhaling completely. Then slowly take a deep breath through your nostrils. There should be a slight sound when you inhale. As you breathe in, contract your abdominal muscles. Fill up your lungs as much as possible. When you have taken in all the air you can, hold your breath for a moment or so. Then exhale slowly and steadily, making sure you completely empty your lungs. You should be able to hear your exhalation. Wait a moment; then inhale again deeply and fully through your nostrils. Repeat complete exercise 10 times.

Breakfast menu (235 calories)
½ grapefruit (48 calories), drizzled with 1 teaspoon honey (21 calories)
1 slice French toast (Open foil package and put frozen toast from Week 1 in
  preheated 400° oven for 10 minutes.) (95 calories)
¼ cup unsweetened applesauce, mixed with ½ teaspoon cinnamon
  (27 calories)
1 4-ounce glass skim milk (44 calories)
Coffee (regular or decaffeinated) or tea (no sugar)

Exercise break: **brisk walk.** Go for a brisk 3-mile walk after breakfast (1½ miles each way), preferably to or in a park.

Daytime

Lunch menu (318 calories)

*Grilled Swiss cheese and tomato sandwich (239 calories)

Tossed green salad made from 2 cups Boston and romaine lettuce leaves, torn into bite-sized pieces (15 calories) and 1 carrot, grated (17 calories); serve with 1 tablespoon low-calorie Italian salad dressing (7 calories)

½ banana (40 calories)

Coffee (regular or decaffeinated) or tea (no sugar or milk)

*Grilled Swiss cheese and tomato sandwich

1 1½-ounce slice Swiss cheese (159 calories)

3 cherry tomatoes, halved (12 calories)

1 slice whole wheat bread (68 calories)

Toast bread lightly and place tomatoes on the bread. Cover with cheese and place 4 inches from flame under broiler. Serve when cheese is melted.

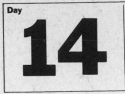
Sunday

Evening

Dinner menu (478 calories)
*1 cup gazpacho (65 calories)
*½ broiled Caribbean chicken breast (164 calories)
½ cup green beans, steamed and sprinkled with dill weed (21 calories)
3 new potatoes, boiled and sprinkled with chopped parsley (92 calories)
1 orange, peeled and sliced in juice from ½ orange and sprinkled with
    cinnamon (92 calories)
Cappuccino (made with ½ cup hot skim milk and ½ cup instant espresso
    coffee, sprinkled with cinnamon) (44 calories)

*Gazpacho
1 8¼-ounce can whole tomatoes
    (50 calories)
½ cucumber, peeled and cut up
    (10 calories)
½ green pepper, seeded and cut up
    (8 calories)

½ onion, chopped (19 calories)
1 clove garlic (3 calories)
1 teaspoon olive oil (40 calories)
2 teaspoons wine vinegar
½ cup cold water

Put tomatoes, cucumber, green pepper, onion, and garlic in the container of an
electric blender. Blend until smooth. Put the tomato mixture into a bowl and add the
olive oil, wine vinegar, and water. Stir to mix thoroughly. Serve very well chilled.
Save ½ for dinner on Day 15.

*Broiled Caribbean chicken breast
1 12-ounce chicken breast, cut in half
    (288 calories)
1 tablespoon fresh lime juice (8 calories)
Juice of ½ orange (32 calories)

½ onion, sliced (19 calories)
1 small bay leaf
¼ teaspoon red pepper sauce

Put chicken in a glass bowl. Combine lime juice, orange juice, onion, bay leaf, and
pepper sauce. Pour over chicken. Marinate for 2 to 3 hours. Place chicken in broiling
pan, 6 inches from flame. (If your broiler pan does not allow for this distance, reduce
the heat.) Broil for about 40 minutes until golden brown. Turn chicken several times
to cook evenly, basting with pan juices. If chicken browns too quickly, decrease heat.
Use ½ for lunch on Day 17.

Last thing before you go to bed: **the tense-and-relaxation technique.** This is a
method of relaxation borrowed from hatha yoga. It is amazingly effective.
Read instructions all the way through before you begin.

Lie on your back on a mat, with feet slightly apart, arms at your side and
palms of hands facing up. Start the exercise by thinking of your toes and
feet. Tense them as tightly as you can and then release the tension. Next,
tense your right leg and release the tension. Do the same with your left leg.
Tense your right arm, clenching your fist, and then release the tension.

Repeat with the left arm and fist. Tense your shoulders and release the tension. Squeeze your lips, eyes, and face together, as though you were going to form a point, and release. Going back to your toes, think about relaxing each toe, the feet, the lower legs, thighs, buttocks, arms, back, the shoulders, the face and scalp, and the back of your neck. Consciously relax every part of your body by letting your soothing thoughts travel up and down.

Eleven o'clock exercise break: mat exercises to relax you and tone your muscles.

Pelvic lift

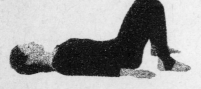

1. Lie on your back, arms at sides and palms down. Bend knees and place feet flat on floor, as close to buttocks as possible.

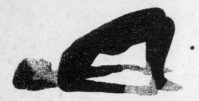

2. Inhaling, raise buttocks and arch back. Hold for a count of 5. Exhaling, return to starting position. Repeat 10 times.

Kneeling leg extension

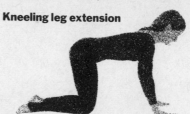

1. Kneel with hands and feet flat on floor.

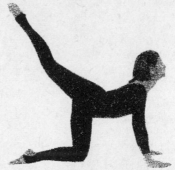

2. Extend right leg back and up as high as is comfortable.

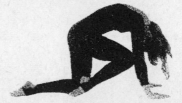

3. Bend knee and bring it forward as close to body as possible, bending head to meet knee. Extend leg back and lift high.

4. Repeat with left leg. Alternate legs 3 times.

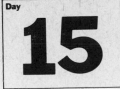

Morning

On arising: **breathing exercise.** Stand by the side of your bed with your spine straight and your feet firmly placed a few inches apart. As you breathe in, lift up your rib cage. Keep your eyes closed while you do the exercise. Concentrate totally on your breathing.

Begin by exhaling completely. Then slowly take a deep breath through your nostrils. There should be a slight sound when you inhale. As you breathe in, contract your abdominal muscles. Fill your lungs as much as possible. When you have taken in all the air you can, hold your breath for a moment or so. Then exhale slowly and steadily, making sure you completely empty your lungs. You should be able to hear your exhalation. Wait a moment; then inhale again deeply and fully through your nostrils. Repeat complete exercise 10 times.

Immediately after breathing exercise: **wake-up exercises.**

Arm circles

1. Stand with feet shoulder width apart. Raise arms to shoulder height. Moving arms forward, make 10 circles in the air.

2. Reverse direction and make 10 more circles.

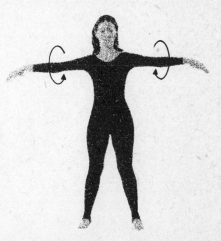

Running in place. Always run on a carpeted or padded surface. Warm up with a slow jog of 40 steps. Rest for a moment and then run at a faster pace for 3 minutes. Cool down by walking around, taking long strides, until your pulse rate and breathing have returned to normal.

Weigh yourself and record your weight.

Breakfast menu (245 calories)
1 4-ounce glass orange juice (55 calories)
1 egg, poached (78 calories)
1 slice whole wheat toast (68 calories)
1 4-ounce glass skim milk (44 calories)
Coffee (regular or decaffeinated) or tea (no sugar)

Brown-bag lunch: If you are taking lunch to your office, prepare it right after breakfast.

"The habit of persistence is the habit of victory."
—HERBERT KAUFMAN

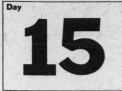

Monday

Daytime

Midmorning break: **herb tea.**

Lunch menu (272 calories)
*Open-faced tuna salad sandwich (227 calories)
½ apple (45 calories)
Coffee (regular or decaffeinated) or tea (no sugar or milk)

*Open-faced tuna salad sandwich

1 3½-ounce can solid white tuna, water-packed (120 calories)
1 tablespoon capers (3 calories)
1 tablespoon parsley, chopped (2 calories)

2 teaspoons diet or imitation mayonnaise (32 calories)
1 leaf romaine lettuce (2 calories)
1 slice whole wheat bread (68 calories)

Combine drained tuna, capers, parsley, and mayonnaise and mix thoroughly. Tear romaine lettuce leaf into small pieces. Cover bread with lettuce, then with the tuna salad.

Midafternoon break: run in place for 1 minute. Enjoy a cup of herb tea after cooling off.

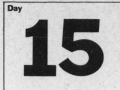
Evening

Dinner menu (520 calories)
1 cup gazpacho (from Day 14) (65 calories)
*Hamburger au poivre, 4 ounces (286 calories)
1 baked potato (Wash, dry, and prick with fork. Bake for 50 minutes in a
   preheated 400° oven.) (90 calories)
Tossed green salad made from 2 cups romaine lettuce leaves, torn into
   bite-sized pieces (15 calories) and sprinkled with 1 tablespoon chopped
   parsley (2 calories); serve with 1 tablespoon low-calorie bleu-cheese salad
   dressing (12 calories)
½ cup green grapes (50 calories)

*Hamburger au poivre

½ pound ground beef round; shape into   1 teaspoon margarine (33 calories)
   two patties and freeze one   1 teaspoon lemon juice (1 calorie)
   (504 calories)   1 dash Worcestershire sauce
1 teaspoon black pepper, cracked   1 dash red pepper sauce
Salt to taste

Heat a nonstick frying pan over high heat and add hamburger. Lower heat to
medium and cook for 3 minutes or until brown. Turn and cook 3 minutes more.
Before serving top burger with melted margarine combined with lemon juice,
Worcestershire sauce, red pepper sauce, salt, and pepper.

Eleven o'clock exercise break: mat exercises to relax you and tone your
muscles.

Seated leg extension

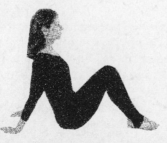
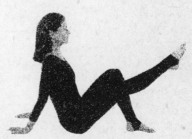

1. Sit with hands placed behind you and   **2.** Extend right leg straight up and then
knees bent.   lower.

                                                3. Repeat with left leg. Alternate, lifting
                                                each leg 3 times.

Kneeling leg extension

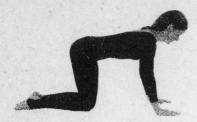

1. Kneel with hands and feet flat on floor.

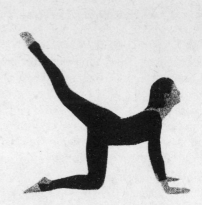

2. Extend right leg back and up as high as is comfortable.

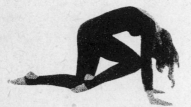

3. Bend knee and bring it forward as close to body as possible, bending head to meet knee. Extend leg back and lift high.

4. Repeat with left leg. Alternate legs 3 times.

Last thing before going to bed: **nature meditation.** Read the exercise all the way through before you start.

Lie flat on your back on a mat. Legs should be slightly separated and relaxed, arms close to your sides, palms of hands facing up. Close your eyes and imagine that you are on an uninhabited tropical island. The sun is high and you can smell the rich fragrance of the flowers. The island is hilly and heavily wooded. Birds screech in the forest. As you climb the hill, you hear a waterfall. The higher you climb, the louder the sound of the water coursing down. Soon you see the falls. The spray catches the sunlight and reflects a brilliant rainbow.

Tuesday

Morning

On arising: **breathing exercise.** Stand by the side of your bed with your spine straight and your feet firmly placed a few inches apart. As you breathe in, lift up your rib cage. Keep your eyes closed while you do the exercise. Concentrate totally on your breathing.

Begin by exhaling completely. Then slowly take a deep breath through your nostrils. There should be a slight sound when you inhale. As you breathe in, contract your abdominal muscles. Fill your lungs as much as possible. When you have taken in all the air you can, hold your breath for a moment or so. Then exhale slowly and steadily, making sure you completely empty your lungs. You should be able to hear your exhalation. Wait a moment; then inhale again deeply and fully through your nostrils. Repeat complete exercise 10 times.

Immediately after breathing exercise: **wake-up exercises.**

Waist circles

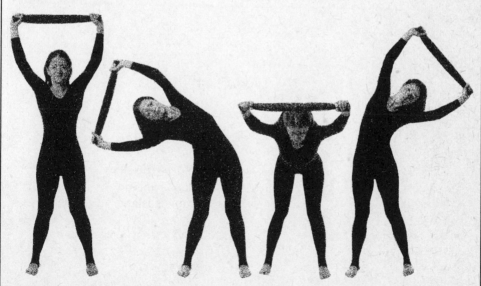

1. Stand with feet shoulder width apart. Holding the ends of a hand towel, lift it overhead with arms straight.

2. Keeping hips centered over feet, bend to the right without straining.

3. Bend forward from the waist, holding the towel straight out in front.

4. Lift arms and bend to the left. Return to starting position. Repeat 10 times.

Running in place. Always run on a carpeted or padded surface. Warm up with a slow jog of 40 steps. Rest for a moment and then run at a faster pace for 3 minutes. Cool down by walking around, taking long strides, until your pulse rate and breathing have returned to normal.

Weigh yourself and record your weight.

Breakfast menu (227 calories)
1 4-ounce glass orange juice (55 calories)
¼ cup cottage cheese, sprinkled with cinnamon, to use as spread for toast (60 calories)
1 slice whole wheat toast (68 calories)
1 4-ounce glass skim milk (44 calories)
Coffee (regular or decaffeinated) or tea (no sugar)

Brown-bag lunch: If you are taking lunch to your office, prepare it right after breakfast.

Note: Transfer frozen flounder fillets from freezer to refrigerator.

Daytime

Midmorning break: **herb tea.**

Lunch menu (224 calories)
*Vegetarian chef's salad (160 calories)
3 melba toast rounds (24 calories)
½ banana (40 calories)
Coffee (regular or decaffeinated) or tea (no sugar or milk)

*Vegetarian chef's salad
1 1-ounce slice Swiss cheese, cut into thin strips (106 calories)
4 cherry tomatoes, halved (16 calories)
1 scallion, thinly sliced (4 calories)
1 carrot, pared into curls (17 calories)

¼ head romaine lettuce, torn into bite-sized pieces (10 calories)
1 tablespoon low-calorie Italian salad dressing (7 calories)

Combine all ingredients and toss with dressing immediately before serving.

Midafternoon break: Run in place for 1 minute. After cooling down, have a cup of herb tea.

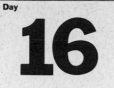

Evening

Dinner menu (501 calories)
*Manhattan fish chowder (301 calories)
Tossed green salad made from 2 cups romaine and Boston lettuce leaves, torn into bite-sized pieces (15 calories); serve with 1 tablespoon lemon-cumin salad dressing (50 calories)
1 breadstick (40 calories)
1 pear (95 calories)
Coffee (regular or decaffeinated) or tea (no sugar or milk)

*Manhattan fish chowder
¼ pound flounder fillet (79 calories)
1 teaspoon margarine (33 calories)
½ onion, chopped (19 calories)
½ green pepper, chopped (8 calories)
1 stalk celery, chopped (5 calories)
1 carrot, chopped (17 calories)

Pinch of thyme
1 8¼-ounce can whole tomatoes (50 calories)
1 potato (90 calories)
1 cup water
1 teaspoon chopped parsley

Melt margarine in a saucepan over medium heat and add onion, green pepper, celery, and carrot. Sauté vegetables for 2 minutes; then add thyme, tomatoes, potato, and ½ cup water and cook for 10 minutes. Add flounder and additional ½ cup water. Cook for another 10 minutes or until fish is done. Serve sprinkled with chopped parsley.

Beauty break: **eyebrows shaped to enhance your face and eyes.** The look of your eyebrows is of great importance to your overall appearance. If the brows are shaped properly to suit your face, your eyes will be more expressive and appealing. Eyebrows that are too heavy or too thin, badly shaped, too dark or too light often detract from your face's good points. Generally, a lighter, lifted brow is more becoming. (The few women who look well with heavy brows usually have unusual eyes.) To achieve the shape that is most becoming to your face requires a little time and study, so set aside enough time to do a really good job, and make eyebrow upkeep a regular part of your beauty program.

You will need: alcohol or witch hazel, cotton pads, old toothbrush (washed thoroughly and dried), a good pair of tweezers, 2 or 3 ice cubes, and medicated moisture lotion.

Your eyebrow should begin directly over the inner corner of your eye. It should arch gently and end about ¼ inch beyond the outer corner of the eye. Use a cotton pad to apply alcohol or witch hazel to the eyebrow area. Next, use the toothbrush to brush your brows up and away from the eye. Study your brows carefully in a mirror to decide which hairs to remove. Generally, it's best to be conservative and first clear out the stray hairs under the arch.

Next, pluck the hairs that extend beyond the inner corner of the eye (toward the nose). Tweeze one hair at a time, plucking in the direction the hair grows, for minimum discomfort. Do not pluck hairs at the top of the brow except for the strays that sometimes grow raggedly at the outer end. If you feel discomfort as you tweeze, apply the ice cube to deaden any pain. After you have achieved a becoming shape, apply the ice cube all along the brow. Dry with a towel and apply a light layer of medicated moisture lotion. Do not use makeup on newly plucked eyebrows. Let the skin rest overnight.

Eleven o'clock exercise break: mat exercises to relax you and tone your muscles.

Kneeling leg extension

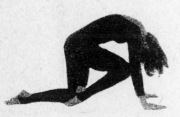

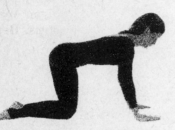

1. Kneel with hands and feet flat on floor.

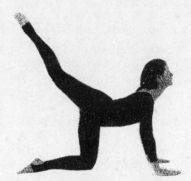

2. Extend right leg back and up as high as is comfortable.

3. Bend knee and bring it forward as close to body as possible, bending head to meet knee. Extend leg back and lift high.

4. Repeat with left leg. Alternate legs 3 times.

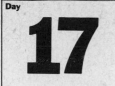
| # Wednesday

Morning

On arising: **breathing exercise.** Stand by the side of your bed with your spine straight and your feet firmly placed a few inches apart. As you breathe in, lift up your rib cage. Keep your eyes closed while you do the exercise. Concentrate totally on your breathing.

Begin by exhaling completely. Then slowly take a deep breath through your nostrils. There should be a slight sound when you inhale. As you breathe in, contract your abdominal muscles. Fill your lungs as much as possible. When you have taken in all the air you can, hold your breath for a moment or so. Then exhale slowly and steadily, making sure you completely empty your lungs. You should be able to hear your exhalation. Wait a moment; then inhale again deeply and fully through your nostrils. Repeat complete exercise 10 times.

Immediately after breathing exercise: **wake-up exercises.**

Hip and side stretch

1. Stand with feet together, left hand on hip and right arm extended straight up.

2. Stretch with your arm over to your left side, then straighten up.

3. Repeat, with right arm above head. Do 10 times to each side.

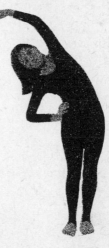

Running in place. Always run on a carpeted or padded surface. Warm up with a slow jog of 50 steps. Rest for a moment and then run at a faster pace for 3 minutes. Cool down by walking around, taking long strides, until your pulse rate and breathing have returned to normal.

Weigh yourself and record your weight.

Breakfast menu (264 calories)
1 4-ounce glass orange juice (55 calories)
¾ cup bran flakes (101 calories)
¼ cup blueberries (20 calories)
1 8-ounce glass skim milk (88 calories)
Coffee (regular or decaffeinated) or tea (no sugar)

Brown-bag lunch: If you are taking lunch to your office, prepare it right after breakfast.

Note: Transfer pork chop from freezer to refrigerator.

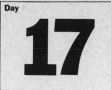

Day 17 | Wednesday

Daytime

Midmorning break: **herb tea.**

Lunch menu (261 calories)
*Slivered chicken salad (181 calories)
1 breadstick (40 calories)
½ banana (40 calories)
Coffee (regular or decaffeinated) or tea (no sugar or milk)

*Slivered chicken salad

½ broiled Caribbean chicken breast
from Day 14, slivered (154 calories)
½ cucumber, peeled and cubed
(10 calories)

4 romaine lettuce leaves, torn into
bite-sized pieces (10 calories)
1 tablespoon low-calorie Italian salad
dressing (7 calories)

Combine all ingredients and toss to mix. If you are taking salad to your office, do not
add dressing until just before lunch.

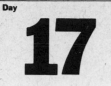
Wednesday

Evening

Dinner menu (489 calories)
*1 orange-baked pork chop (245 calories)
*1 cup lemon-glazed carrots (58 calories)
1 zucchini, cut in rounds and steamed (26 calories) and sprinkled with 1
   chopped scallion (4 calories)
Tossed green salad made from 2 cups romaine lettuce leaves, torn into
   bite-sized pieces (15 calories) and 4 cherry tomatoes, halved (16 calories);
   serve with 1 tablespoon low-calorie Italian salad dressing (7 calories)
½ cup coffee yogurt (100 calories), sprinkled with 1 tablespoon roasted,
   slivered almonds (18 calories)

*Orange-baked pork chop

1 4-ounce pork chop (3 ounces meat)   ¼ teaspoon poultry seasoning
  (231 calories)   Pinch salt
2 tablespoons orange juice (14 calories)   Black pepper, freshly ground

Brown chop quickly in a nonstick frying pan; then transfer to a small baking dish.
Pour orange juice over chop, sprinkle on poultry seasoning, salt, and pepper. Bake,
covered, in a preheated 400° oven for 30 minutes, or until chop is done.

*Lemon-glazed carrots

2 medium carrots, cut in rounds   1 teaspoon honey (21 calories)
  (34 calories)   1 tablespoon lemon juice (3 calories)
½ cup water   Grated rind of ½ lemon
Pinch salt

Put water and salt in a small saucepan and bring to a boil. Add carrots and simmer,
covered, for 10 to 12 minutes. Drain. Combine honey, lemon juice, lemon rind and
mix thoroughly. Pour lemon-honey mixture over carrots and stir to mix.

Eleven o'clock exercise break: mat exercises to relax you and tone your
muscles.

Seated extended stretch

Leg lift

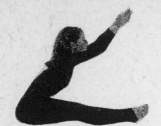

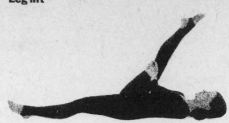

1. Sit with lets together straight out in front of you. Lift arms to meet above head, palms together.

2. Bend down keeping spine straight, arms extended, and legs flat on floor.

1. Lie on your back, legs straight out in front of you and arms at your sides. Lift right leg without bending knee.

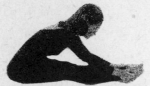

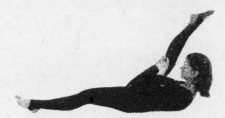

3. Grasp ankles with hands and holds for a count of 5. Return to starting position. Repeat 5 times.

2. With both hands, grasp leg behind knee and lift head to meet knee. Hold for a count of 3. Slowly return to starting position.

3. Repeat with left leg. Alternate, lifting each leg 5 times.

Last thing before you go to bed: **relaxation technique.** Read through the exercise before you start.

Lie down on your back on the mat, with your legs separated and relaxed and your arms close to your sides, with the palms of your hands facing up. This exercise will be a repeat of the exercise in which you move up the body from your toes to the top of your head with your mind's eye, progressively replacing each part of your body. Close your eyes and take several deep breaths. With your mind focused on your right big toe, relax the muscles of that toe; move from toe to toe, then up the foot around to the bottom of the foot, up the ankle, the shin, the knee, the thigh. Cover every inch of muscle in your body. Do your left foot and leg. Move up to the pubic area and around to the buttocks. Go back, up over the abdomen, up the rib cage, the neck, and face. Do the whole head, moving slowly over the top of the head, down the back to the nape of the neck and the shoulders. Spend a little extra time on the shoulder area because sedentary people often get especially tense there. Move down the back until you reach the tip of the spine. When you have finished, lie still for a few moments and concentrate on your breathing.

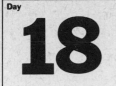

Thursday

Morning

On arising: **breathing exercise.** Stand by the side of your bed with your spine straight and your feet firmly placed a few inches apart. As you breathe in, lift up your rib cage. Keep your eyes closed while you do the exercise. Concentrate totally on your breathing.

Begin by exhaling completely. Then slowly take a deep breath through your nostrils. There should be a slight sound when you inhale. As you breathe in, contract your abdominal muscles. Fill your lungs as much as possible. When you have taken in all the air you can, hold your breath for a moment. Then exhale slowly and steadily, making sure you completely empty your lungs. You should be able to hear your exhalation. Wait a moment; then inhale again deeply and fully through your nostrils. Repeat complete exercise 10 times.

Immediately after breathing exercise: **wake-up exercises.**

Waist circles

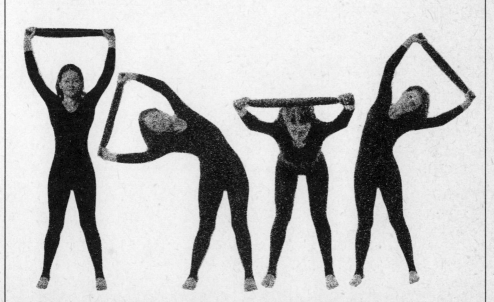

1. Stand with feet shoulder width apart. Holding the ends of a hand towel, lift it overhead with arms straight.

2. Keeping hips centered over feet, bend to the right without straining.

3. Bend forward from the waist, holding the towel straight out in front.

4. Lift arms and bend to the left. Return to starting position. Repeat 10 times.

Running in place. Always run on a carpeted or padded surface. Warm up by jogging very slowly for 50 steps. Rest for a moment and then run at a faster pace for 3½ minutes. Cool down by walking around, taking long strides, until your pulse rate and breathing have returned to normal.

Weigh yourself and record your weight.

Breakfast menu (238 calories)
½ grapefruit (48 calories)
1 egg, scrambled in nonstick pan (78 calories)
1 slice whole wheat toast (68 calories)
1 4-ounce glass skim milk (44 calories)
Coffee (regular or decaffeinated) or tea (no sugar)

Brown-bag lunch: If you are taking lunch to your office, prepare it right after breakfast.

Note: Transfer boneless chicken breast from freezer to refrigerator.

"It is easier to suppress the first desire than to satisfy all that follow it."
—BENJAMIN FRANKLIN

Daytime

Midmorning break: **herb tea.**

Lunch menu (303 calories)
*Fruit and cottage cheese salad (279 calories)
3 melba toast rounds (24 calories)
Coffee (regular or decaffeinated) or tea (no sugar or milk)

*Fruit and cottage cheese salad
½ cup cottage cheese (120 calories)
¼ apple, cored and cut into cubes
  (45 calories)
½ orange, peeled and sliced (32 calories)
¼ cup vanilla yogurt (50 calories)

1 tablespoon toasted wheat germ
  (27 calories)
2 leaves romaine lettuce, torn into
  bite-sized pieces (5 calories)

Place cottage cheese on bed of lettuce. Cover with fruit and then yogurt. Sprinkle wheat germ over all.

Midafternoon break: Run in place for 1 minute. After cooling off, have a cup of herb tea.

Evening

Dinner menu (444 calories)
*Chicken yakitori (169 calories)
½ cup cooked white rice (112 calories)
Tossed green salad made from 2 cups romaine and Boston lettuce leaves, torn into bite-sized pieces (15 calories), ½ cucumber, peeled and sliced (10 calories), 4 radishes, sliced (7 calories), and 1 carrot, shaved into curls (17 calories); serve with 1 tablespoon lemon-cumin salad dressing (50 calories)
1 orange, peeled and sliced (64 calories)
Coffee (regular or decaffeinated) or tea (no sugar or milk)

*Chicken yakitori

1 6-ounce boneless chicken breast (144 calories)
½ clove garlic, finely chopped (1 calorie)
2 tablespoons soy sauce (20 calories)
2 tablespoons lemon juice (6 calories)
½ teaspoon sugar (7 calories)
2 scallions, cut into 2-inch pieces (8 calories)

Remove skin from chicken breast and cut meat into 1-inch squares. In small bowl, combine garlic, soy sauce, lemon juice, and sugar. Add chicken squares to soy-sauce mixture and stir to coat evenly. Cover bowl with plastic wrap. Marinate for about 1 hour. Thread chicken onto small skewers, with a piece of scallion between chicken sections. Broil 4 inches from flame for about 3 minutes. Remove from broiler, baste with marinade, and broil on other side for 2 to 3 minutes more or until chicken is done.

Beauty break: **eye makeup—part 1.** Well-applied eye makeup can create beautiful eyes, but poorly applied makeup is worse than none at all. It takes thought and practice to learn what is right for you. Generally speaking, the brightest colors and frosted shadows are the most difficult to wear. Bright blues, greens, and turquoises usually look harsh and too obvious; because they are so bright, they usually overwhelm the eyes they are meant to enhance. There are many beautiful muted shades to choose from, and these quieter colors are much more flattering to eyes and skin tones than the stronger ones. To get good ideas of what might be suitable for you, study fashion magazines. Also, study your eyes in bright sunlight. Many times the iris of the eye is a blend of colors, and you may discover a shade that will intensify your eye color when used on your eyelids.

You will need: a good magnifying hand mirror and two or three muted shades of powdered eye shadow.

For the daytime, eye shadow looks best when it is applied to the lid and not above the crease or on the brow bone. Highlighters tend to look garish by day and are more effective at night. Even at night never use a stark white highlighter.

After you have applied eye shadow on the lid, you might like to try extending it a little beyond the corner of the eye—this will be especially appealing if you are using a taupe, fawn-brown, or gray shade. Then draw a thin line of shadow under the lower lashes, starting at the center of the eye and extending to the outer corner. If you like, you can use a slightly darker shade in the crease of the eye. Or, try using a gray or brown shade in the crease and as an eyeliner. This is a practice session to see what it is most becoming to you.

Eleven o'clock exercise break: mat exercises to relax you and tone your muscles.

Leg lift

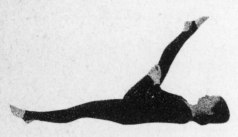

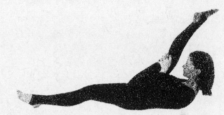

1. Lie on your back, legs straight out in front of you and arms at your sides. Lift right leg without bending knee.

2. With both hands, grasp leg behind knee and lift head to meet knee. Hold for a count of 3. Slowly return to starting position.

3. Repeat with left leg. Alternate, lifting each leg 5 times.

Friday

Morning

On arising: **breathing exercise.** Stand by the side of your bed with your spine straight and your feet firmly placed a few inches apart. As you breathe in, lift up your rib cage. Keep your eyes closed while you do the exercise. Concentrate totally on your breathing.

Begin by exhaling completely. Then slowly take a deep breath through your nostrils. There should be a slight sound when you inhale. As you breathe in, contract your abdominal muscles. Fill up your lungs as much as possible. When you have taken in all the air you can, hold your breath for a moment or so. Then exhale slowly and steadily, making sure you completely empty your lungs. You should be able to hear your exhalation. Wait a moment; then inhale again deeply and fully through your nostrils. Repeat complete exercise 10 times.

Immediately after breathing exercise: **wake-up exercises.**

Leg swing

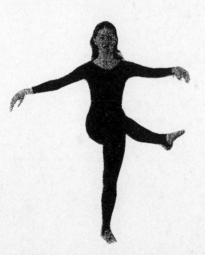

1. Stand with feet 6 inches apart. Lift arms to shoulder height, palms facing down.

2. Swing left leg up in front and then to the right at hip level. Return to starting position.

3. Swing right leg up and to the left. Repeat 10 times.

Running in place. Always run on a carpeted or padded surface. Warm up by jogging very slowly for 50 steps. Rest for a moment and then run at a faster pace for 3½ minutes. Cool down by walking around, taking long strides, until your pulse rate and breathing have returned to normal.

Weigh yourself and record your weight.

Breakfast menu (230 calories)
½ grapefruit (48 calories)
¼ cup pineapple cottage cheese, to use as a spread on toast (70 calories)
1 slice whole wheat toast (68 calories)
1 4-ounce glass skim milk (44 calories)
Coffee (regular or decaffeinated) or tea (no sugar)

Brown-bag lunch: If you are taking lunch to your office, prepare it right after breakfast.

Note: Transfer veal scaloppine from freezer to refrigerator.

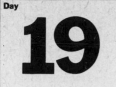

Daytime

Midmorning break: **herb tea**

Lunch menu (277 calories)
*Spinach and tuna salad (198 calories)
1 breadstick (40 calories)
1 tangerine (39 calories)
Coffee (regular or decaffeinated) or tea (no sugar or milk)

*Spinach and tuna salad

½ pound fresh spinach, washed, dried, and stems removed (44 calories)

1 3½-ounce can solid white tuna, water-packed (120 calories)

4 cherry tomatoes, halved (16 calories)

1 scallion, thinly sliced (4 calories)

2 tablespoons low-calorie Italian salad dressing (14 calories)

Tear spinach leaves into bite-sized pieces. Combine all ingredients. Toss with dressing immediately before serving.

Midafternoon break: Run in place for 1 minute. After cooling off, have a cup of herb tea.

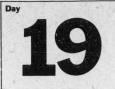

Evening

Dinner menu (491 calories)
*Veal piccata (288 calories)
1 cup cooked noodles (100 calories)
Tossed green salad made from 2 cups romaine and Boston lettuce leaves,
    torn into bite-sized pieces (15 calories); serve with 1 tablespoon
    low-calorie bleu-cheese salad dressing (12 calories)
½ cup strawberries (26 calories) in ¼ cup vanilla yogurt (50 calories)
Coffee (regular or decaffeinated) or tea (no sugar or milk)

*Veal Piccata
¼ pound veal scaloppine (247 calories)
1 teaspoon margarine (33 calories)
2 teaspoons lemon juice (6 calories)
2 tablespoons chicken stock, made from
    bouillon cube

Pinch of salt
Pinch of pepper
1 tablespoon parsley, chopped (2
    calories)
2 thin slices lemon

Pound veal slices thin with a mallet. Cut into pieces about 1½ inches square. Put margarine in nonstick frying pan over medium-high heat. When margarine is melted, add veal and brown on both sides. Add lemon juice, chicken stock, salt, pepper, and parsley. Cook gently for 2 minutes longer. Serve garnished with thin slices of lemon.

Eleven o'clock exercise break: mat exercises to relax you and tone your muscles.

Reverse leg lifts

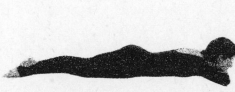
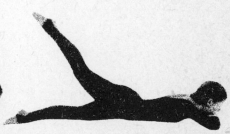

1. Lie on your stomach, arms bent at elbows and chin resting on hands.

2. Keeping it straight, lift right leg straight up as high as possible. Hold for a count of 5.

3. Repeat with left leg. Alternate, lifting each leg 5 times.

Pelvic twist with extended legs

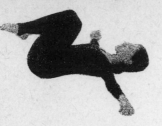
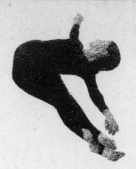

1. Lie on your back, arms out at shoulder level. Inhaling, raise both knees and bring as close to body as possible.

2. Roll to the right, straightening legs. Lower legs to floor. Bring legs back to center bent position. Repeat, rolling to the left. Roll to each side 3 times.

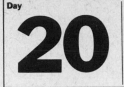

Saturday

Morning

On arising: **breathing exercise.** Stand by the side of your bed with your spine straight and your feet firmly placed a few inches apart. As you breathe in, lift up your rib cage. Keep your eyes closed while you do the exercise. Concentrate totally on your breathing.

Begin by exhaling completely. Then slowly take a deep breath through your nostrils. There should be a slight sound when you inhale. As you breathe in, contract your abdominal muscles. Fill your lungs as much as possible. When you have taken in all the air you can, hold your breath for a moment or so. Then exhale slowly and steadily, making sure you completely empty your lungs. You should be able to hear your exhalation. Wait a moment; then inhale again deeply and fully through your nostrils. Repeat complete exercise 10 times.

Immediately after breathing exercise: **wake-up exercises.**

Overhead arm swing

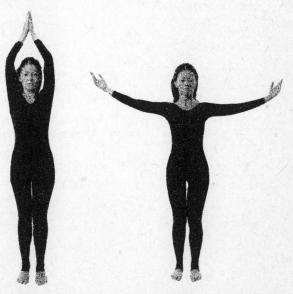

1. Stand with feet together. Lift up on toes, breathing in and raising arms until palms meet overhead.

2. Breathe out as you lower heels to floor and bring arms down to your sides. Repeat 10 times.

Running in place. Always run on a carpeted or padded surface. Warm up by jogging very slowly for 50 steps. Rest for a moment and then run at a faster pace for 3½ minutes. Cool down by walking around, taking long strides, until your pulse rate and breathing have returned to normal.

Weigh yourself and record your weight.

Breakfast menu (249 calories)
1 4-ounce glass orange juice (55 calories)
1 slice French toast (Open foil package and put frozen toast from Week 1 in preheated 400° oven for 10 minutes.) (95 calories)
½ cup unsweetened applesauce, mixed with ½ teaspoon cinnamon (55 calories)
1 4-ounce glass skim milk (44 calories)
Coffee (regular or decaffeinated) or tea (no sugar)

Shopping List

Breads
1 package hamburger buns (freeze whatever is not used)

Dairy products
1 12-ounce container cottage cheese
1 8-ounce container pineapple cottage cheese
1 dozen medium eggs

Fruits and vegetables
2 2½-inch apples
2 7-inch bananas
1 4-inch grapefruit
1 quart orange juice
1 3-inch orange
2 3-inch pears
2 2½-inch tangerines
1 10-ounce package frozen asparagus
1 bunch carrots
1 7-inch cucumber
¼ pound medium mushrooms (about 8)
1 bunch parsley
1 head Boston lettuce
1 head romaine lettuce
1 1-pint carton cherry tomatoes
1 3-inch tomato
1 8-ounce can tomato sauce
2 bunches radishes
1 6-inch zucchini
1 3-ounce green pepper
1 bunch scallions
1 baking potato (about ¼ pound)
1 pound potatoes (3 to a pound)

Meat and fish
½ pound ground lamb (store in freezer)
1 4-ounce minute steak
1 6-ounce veal chop
1 12-ounce chicken breast
1 3½-ounce can solid white tuna, water-packed

Other items
1 11-ounce bottle mineral water
1 4-ounce can walnut halves
1 8-ounce bottle low-calorie Italian salad dressing

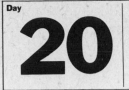

Day 20 | # Saturday

Daytime

Lunch menu (279 calories)
*Grilled ham and cheese sandwich (235 calories)
4 radishes (7 calories)
1 stalk celery (5 calories)
½ orange (32 calories)
Coffee (regular or decaffeinated) or tea (no sugar or milk)

*Grilled ham and cheese sandwish
1 slice whole wheat bread (68 calories)
1 1-ounce slice boiled ham (53 calories)
1 1-ounce slice Swiss cheese (106 calories)
1 teaspoon mustard (8 calories)

Lightly toast the bread and spread on mustard. Place ham slice and then cheese slice on the bread. Place under broiler until cheese melts.

Beauty break: **eye makeup—part 2.** Since the days of Cleopatra and the early temple paintings in India, women have known that eye makeup increases the beauty of their eyes. But it takes practice and skill to do it well (as it does most other things), and it's also important to use the right equipment and products. Today many women wear a smudgy or muted eyeliner and mascara during the day, using shadows only at night. If you do this, it's important to learn to apply liner so that it does not have a harsh look and to apply mascara in thin enough coats so that you do not have clumpy-looking or spiky eyelashes. Also, curling your lashes with an eyelash curler is a basic step to more beautiful eyes.

You will need: eyelash curler, brown, gray, or black eyeliner, and cake or roll-on mascara.

Whatever form of eyeliner you use, remember that you are trying for a smudgy, soft line as close to the lashes as possible. After applying, take a tightly rolled cotton swab or a fairly firm makeup brush and soften the line by smudging it gently. With practice, you will be able to achieve exactly the look you want. Try doing your lower lashes as well. The now-popular blue line above the lower lashes looks too made-up for day and should be reserved for evening makeup. Next, curl your lashes with the eyelash curler. This makes the lashes seem longer and fuller and gives the eye a more open look. It only takes a few minutes, and it's much more effective than false eyelashes, which should be reserved for actresses and other performers. Now you are ready to apply mascara. Very pale blondes and redheads can use brown, everyone else looks best with black or black-brown mascara. Apply at least two coats to get the thick-lashed look. Let the first coat dry before applying the second, using an old toothbrush or a makeup brush to remove extra mascara and make sure lashes stay separated. Apply the second coat and brush again.

Beauty break checklist for upcoming week

Mild soap

Pumice stone

Body lotion

Nail polish remover

Cotton pads

Nail clippers

Emery board

Cuticle remover

Orangewood stick

Facial tissues

Nail polish

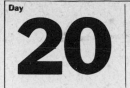

Evening

Dinner menu (482 calories)
1 11-ounce glass mineral water with ice and a thin slice of lemon
*Minute steak with mushrooms (281 calories)
*½ stuffed baked potato (60 calories)
Tossed green salad made from ¼ head Boston lettuce, torn into bite-sized
 pieces (6 calories), 4 cherry tomatoes, halved (16 calories), and 1 carrot,
 cut into curls (17 calories); serve with 1 tablespoon low-calorie Italian
 salad dressing (7 calories)
1 pear (95 calories)
Coffee (regular or decaffeinated) or tea (no sugar or milk)

*Minute steak with mushrooms
1 4-ounce minute steak (236 calories)
1 teaspoon Worcestershire sauce
1 tablespoon soy sauce (10 calories)
2 scallions, thinly sliced (8 calories)

⅓ cup beef broth, made from bouillon
 cube (2 calories)
5 mushrooms, sliced (25 calories)

Combine Worcestershire sauce, soy sauce, scallions, and half the broth in a bowl.
Marinate steak in this mixture for 1 hour. Heat a nonstick frying pan over high heat.
Remove steak from marinade, dry on paper towel, and put into hot pan to brown.
Cook for 2 minutes and turn to cook on other side for 2 minutes. Remove steak from
pan and keep warm. Reduce heat to medium-high, put mushrooms in pan, and cook
for 2 minutes. Turn mushrooms and add marinade and remaining beef broth. Simmer
for 2 to 3 minutes. Pour mushroom sauce over steak and serve.

*Stuffed baked potato
1 baking potato, scrubbed, pricked with
 a fork (90 calories)
2 tablespoons skim milk, heated (11
 calories)

1 tablespoon Parmesan cheese, grated
 (20 calories)
Salt
Pepper
Paprika

Preheat oven to 425°. Place potato on a rack in oven and bake for 45 to 60 minutes or
until tender when tested with a fork. When potato is still hot but cool enough to
handle, cut it into halves and scoop out the inside, leaving just enough potato to form
a shell. Mash the potato well and add heated milk, salt, pepper, and cheese. Stir well
to blend. Spoon the potato mixture back into the shells and sprinkle with paprika.
Put one potato half in a small baking pan and return to the oven for several minutes
until heated through. Refrigerate other half for use on Day 22.

Eleven o'clock exercise break: mat exercises to relax you and tone your muscles.

Seated body stretch

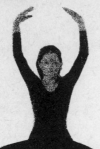

1. Sit with legs wide apart. Lift arms straight up, palms turned inward.

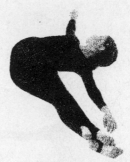

2. Stretch as far to the right side as is comfortable. Return to starting position.

3. Stretch over to the left side. Repeat 5 times to each side.

Pelvic twist with extended legs

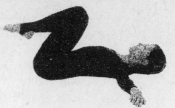

1. Lie on your back, arms out at shoulder level. Inhaling, raise both knees and bring as close to body as possible.

2. Roll to the right, straightening legs. Lower legs to floor. Bring legs back to center bent position. Repeat, rolling to the left. Roll to each side 3 times.

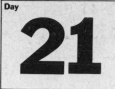

Morning

On arising: **breathing exercise.** Stand by the side of your bed with your spine straight and your feet firmly placed a few inches apart. As you breathe in, lift up your rib cage. Keep your eyes closed while you do the exercise. Concentrate totally on your breathing.

Begin by exhaling completely. Then slowly take a deep breath through your nostrils. There should be a slight sound when you inhale. As you breathe in, contract your abdominal muscles. Fill your lungs as much as possible. When you have taken in all the air you can, hold your breath for a moment or so. Then exhale slowly and steadily, making sure you completely empty your lungs. You should be able to hear your exhalation. Wait a moment; then inhale again deeply and fully through your nostrils. Repeat complete exercise 10 times.

Immediately after breathing exercise: **wake-up exercises.**

Leg swing

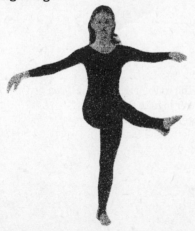
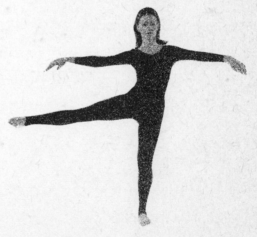

1. Stand with feet 6 inches apart. Lift arms to shoulder height, palms facing down.

2. Swing left leg up in front and then to the right at hip level. Return to starting position.

3. Swing right leg up and to the left. Repeat 10 times.

Breakfast menu (293 calories)
1 4-ounce glass orange juice (55 calories)
*Mushroom omelet (126 calories)
1 slice whole wheat toast (68 calories)
1 4-ounce glass skim milk (44 calories)
Coffee (regular or decaffeinated) or tea (no sugar)

*Mushroom omelet

1 egg (78 calories)
1 teaspoon water
3 fresh mushrooms, sliced
(15 calories)

1 teaspoon margarine (33 calories)
¼ teaspoon marjoram
Freshly ground black pepper to taste

Add 1 teaspoon water to egg and beat just enough to mix. Melt margarine in small frying pan over medium heat. Add sliced mushrooms and sauté lightly. Sprinkle mushrooms with marjoram and pepper. Heat small nonstick frying pan over high heat. Pour in egg and tilt to spread it over the surface of the pan. When egg is nearly cooked, place mushrooms over half of the eggs. With a spatula, gently flip the other half of the egg over the mushrooms. Tilt pan to slide omelet off onto a platter.

Daytime

Midmorning break: Go for a 3-mile walk, inviting a friend to come along.

Lunch menu (231 calories)
*Fruit and cottage cheese salad (207 calories)
3 melba toast rounds (24 calories)
Coffee (regular or decaffeinated) or tea (no sugar or milk)

*Fruit and cottage cheese salad
½ cup cottage cheese (120 calories)
½ apple, cored and cut into cubes
  (45 calories)

½ orange, peeled and cut into cubes
  (32 calories)
4 leaves romaine lettuce, torn into
  bite-sized pieces (10 calories)

Place cottage cheese on bed of lettuce and surround with fruit.

Evening

Dinner menu (493 calories)
*½ chicken cacciatore (227 calories)
1 potato, boiled in its jacket (90 calories)
Tossed green salad made from 2 cups romaine and Boston lettuce leaves,
   torn into bite-sized pieces (15 calories), 1 tablespoon parsley, chopped
   (2 calories), and 4 radishes, sliced (7 calories); serve with 1 tablespoon
   low-calorie bleu-cheese salad dressing (12 calories)
½ cup coffee yogurt (100 calories), sprinkled with ¼ teaspoon cinnamon and 1
   tablespoon chopped walnuts (40 calories)
Coffee (regular, or instant espresso with lemon peel) or tea (no sugar or
   milk)

*Chicken cacciatore

1 12-ounce chicken breast, cut in half (288 calories)
1 teaspoon margarine (33 calories)
1 can (8-ounces) tomato sauce (80 calories)
1 onion, chopped (38 calories)
1 clove garlic, minced (3 calories)
1 stalk celery, chopped (5 calories)

½ green pepper, seeded and chopped (8 calories)
¼ teaspoon oregano
¼ teaspoon basil
1 bay leaf
⅓ cup chicken broth, made from chicken bouillon cube (2 calories)

Melt margarine in a nonstick frying pan over high heat. When pan is hot, brown
chicken on both sides. Remove chicken and place in a flameproof casserole. Put
onion, garlic, celery, and green pepper in frying pan and sauté for 1 minute. Add
tomato sauce and simmer for 2 minutes. Add oregano, basil, bay leaf, and chicken
broth to tomato sauce. Stir to mix thoroughly. Pour sauce over chicken and bring to a
boil. Cover and lower heat. Simmer for 45 minutes. Serve half the breast and sauce
tonight. Reserve other half for dinner on Day 23.

Eleven o'clock exercise break: mat exercises to relax you and tone your
muscles.

Seated extended stretch

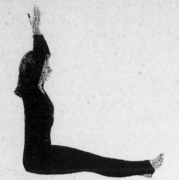

1. Sit with legs together straight out in front of you. Lift arms to meet above head, palms together.

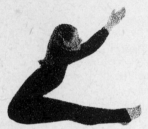

2. Bend down keeping spine straight, arms extended, and legs flat on floor.

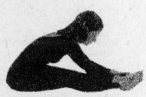

3. Grasp ankles with hands and hold for a count of 5. Return to starting position. Repeat 5 times.

Roll ups

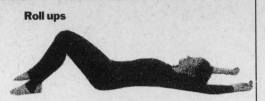

1. Lie on your back, arms extended above your head. Have knees bent and feet flat on floor.

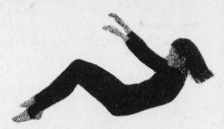

2. Inhaling, slowly rise up to a sitting position.

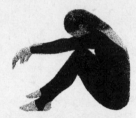

3. Stretch forward with your arms, touching your feet or shins. Exhaling, slowly return to starting position. Repeat 10 times.

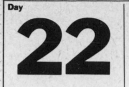

Morning

On arising: **breathing exercise.** Stand by the side of your bed with feet together, spine erect, and shoulders relaxed. Begin by exhaling completely. Take in a deep breath through the nostrils. Try to fill your lungs to capacity. Hold breath for a moment. Exhale slowly and steadily, making a humming sound as you do so. Empty lungs completely. Wait a moment and then repeat exercise. Do 10 inhalations and exhalations.

After breathing exercises: **wake-up exercises.**

Hip and side stretch

1. Stand with feet together, left hand on hip and right arm extended straight up.

2. Stretch with your arm over to your left side, then straighten up.

3. Repeat, with right arm above head. Do 10 times to each side.

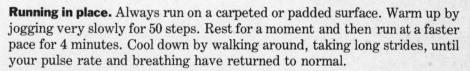

Running in place. Always run on a carpeted or padded surface. Warm up by jogging very slowly for 50 steps. Rest for a moment and then run at a faster pace for 4 minutes. Cool down by walking around, taking long strides, until your pulse rate and breathing have returned to normal.

Weigh yourself and record your weight.

Breakfast menu (230 calories)
½ grapefruit (48 calories)
¼ cup pineapple cottage cheese, to use as spread on toast (70 calories)
1 slice whole wheat toast (68 calories)
1 4-ounce glass skim milk (44 calories)
Coffee (regular or decaffeinated) or tea (no sugar)

Brown-bag lunch: If you are taking lunch to your office, prepare it right after breakfast.

"Without discipline there's no life at all."
—KATHARINE HEPBURN

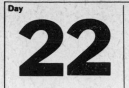

Day
22 | Monday

Daytime

Midmorning break: **herb tea.**

Lunch menu (252 calories)
*Tuna salad (196 calories)
2 melba toast rounds (16 calories)
½ banana (40 calories)
Coffee (regular or decaffeinated) or tea (no sugar or milk)

*Tuna salad
1 3½-ounce can solid white tuna, water-packed (120 calories)

¼ head romaine lettuce, torn into bite-sized pieces (10 calories)

3 cherry tomatoes, halved (12 calories)

1 scallion, thinly sliced (4 calories)

1 tablespoon lemon-cumin salad dressing (50 calories)

Toss all ingredients together to mix thoroughly. If you are taking salad to your office, keep dressing separate and pour on just before eating.

Midafternoon break: Stand erect and take 5 deep breaths. Run in place for 1 minute. Have a cup of herb tea after cooling off.

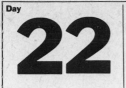
Monday

Evening

Dinner menu (495 calories)
*Broiled veal chop with lemon and rosemary (332 calories)
½ stuffed baked potato (from Day 20) (60 calories)
6 asparagus spears (Use a 10-ounce package of frozen asparagus spears. Cook according to package directions. Reserve remaining asparagus for dinner on Day 23.) (18 calories)
½ cucumber (10 calories), 5 cherry tomatoes (20 calories), and one stalk celery (5 calories), chopped together and sprinkled with 1 scallion, thinly sliced (4 calories); serve with 1 tablespoon low-calorie Italian salad dressing (7 calories)
1 tangerine (39 calories)
Coffee (regular or decaffeinated) or tea (no sugar or milk)

*Broiled veal chop with lemon and rosemary
1 6-ounce veal chop (330 calories)
1 tablespoon lemon juice (3 calories)
¼ teaspoon rosemary
Marinate veal chop in lemon juice and rosemary for ½ hour. Broil 4 inches from flame for 8 minutes on each side or until done.

Eleven o'clock exercise break: mat exercises to relax you and tone your muscles.

Pelvic lift

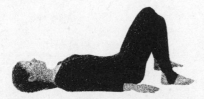 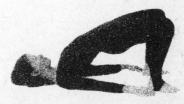

1. Lie on your back, arms at sides and palms down. Bend knees and place feet flat on floor, as close to buttocks as possible.

2. Inhaling, raise buttocks and arch back. Hold for a count of 5. Exhaling, return to starting position. Repeat 10 times.

Knee lift

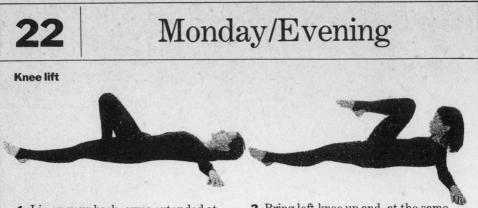

1. Lie on your back, arms extended at shoulder level.

2. Bring left knee up and, at the same time, lift head so that forehead reaches toward knee.

3. Repeat with right knee. Alternate knees, bringing each knee up 10 times.

Last thing before going to bed: nature meditation. Read the exercise all the way through before you start.

Lie flat on a mat, with your legs slightly separated and relaxed and your arms by your sides, palms facing up. Close your eyes and imagine a gently curving white sand beach on a Caribbean island. It is shaded by coconut palms. As you walk along the beach you look out on a small sheltered bay. The water is a brilliant palette of blue, turquoise, and green. You sit beside one of the palm trees, rest your back against its trunk, and gaze out at the water and the bright blue, cloudless sky. A sailboat glides into view. Relax and enjoy the warmth and beauty.

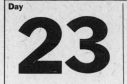
23 | Tuesday

Morning

On arising: **breathing exercise.** Stand by the side of your bed with feet together, spine erect, and shoulders relaxed. Begin by exhaling completely. Take in a deep breath through the nostrils. Try to fill your lungs to capacity. Hold breath for a moment. Exhale slowly and steadily, making a humming sound as you do so. Empty lungs completely. Wait a moment and then repeat exercise. Do 10 inhalations and exhalations.

After breathing exercises: **wake-up exercises.**

Hip and side stretch

1. Stand with feet together, left hand on hip and right arm extended straight up.

2. Stretch with your arm over to your left side, then straighten up.

3. Repeat, with right arm above head. Do 10 times to each side.

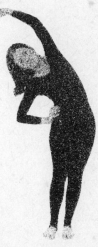

Running in place. Always run on a carpeted or padded surface. Warm up by jogging very slowly for 50 steps. Rest for a moment and then run at a faster pace, lifting feet 4 inches from the floor. Run for 4 minutes. Cool down by walking around, taking long strides, until your pulse rate and breathing have returned to normal.

Weigh yourself and record your weight.

Breakfast menu (238 calories)
½ grapefruit (48 calories)
1 egg, soft-cooked (78 calories)
1 slice whole wheat toast (68 calories)
1 4-ounce glass skim milk (44 calories)
Coffee (regular or decaffeinated) or tea (no sugar)

Brown-bag lunch: If you are taking lunch to your office, prepare it right after breakfast.

Tuesday

Daytime

Midmorning break: **herb tea.**

Lunch menu (245 calories)
*Peanut butter and banana sandwich (201 calories)
1 4-ounce glass skim milk (44 calories)
Coffee (regular or decaffeinated) or tea (no sugar or milk)

*Peanut butter and banana sandwich
1 slice whole wheat bread (68 calories)
1 tablespoon peanut butter (93 calories)
½ banana (40 calories)
Spread bread with peanut butter and top with banana slices.

Midafternoon break: Stand erect and shake hands and arms vigorously. Run in place for 1 minute. After cooling off, relax with coffee or tea.

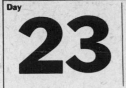
23 | Tuesday

Evening

Dinner menu (503 calories)
½ chicken cacciatore (Reheat remainder from dinner on Day 21.)
   (227 calories)
½ cup cooked white rice (112 calories)
2 romaine lettuce leaves, torn into bite-sized pieces (5 calories) and 6 cooked,
   chilled asparagus spears (18 calories), drizzled with 1 tablespoon low-
   calorie Italian salad dressing (7 calories)
1 apple (90 calories)
Cappuccino (made with ½ cup instant espresso and ½ cup hot skim milk,
   sprinkled with cinnamon) (44 calories)

Beauty break: **how to have beautiful, healthy feet—Part 1.** Healthy, well-cared-for feet are good to look at, and they are also essential for correct posture and an overall feeling of comfort. If your feet feel good, you feel good. There are two parts to a sensible foot-care program. One consists of massage and exercise, and the other is a systematic twice-monthly pedicure. If you follow the system presented here, your feet will be in much better shape, and you may very well improve your state of mind. Part 1 appears here. Part 2 will be done on Thursday evening.

You will need: a basin large enough to accommodate your feet, mild soap, washcloth, pumice stone, body lotion, a book about 2 inches thick, and a pencil.

Fill basin with warm water. Add soap, washcloth, and pumice stone. Soak your feet for 5 minutes in the water; then scrub them with the soapy washcloth. Next, use the pumice stone on any rough or calloused areas. Press firmly, using a circular motion. When you have achieved the knack of using just the right amount of pressure, you will know it! There is a pleasant, rather than abrasive, sensation. This treatment is very effective for scrubbing away dead and toughened skin. When you have done a thorough job with the pumice, rinse your feet in cool water and dry them with a towel. Apply body lotion, and as you do so, give your feet a thorough massage. Begin by taking each toe and rotating it around in a circle. Then take your ankle in one hand and the ball of your foot in the other. Press them gently in opposite directions. Next, pull each toe gently away from the one next to it. Finally, go over the entire foot, from toes to ankles, kneading gently with the fingers of both hands.

Stand up and shake each foot vigorously. Then stand with your feet together and do the following exercises:

1. Raise up on toes; lower heels to floor. Do this 10 times.

2. Next, put the book down in front of you and place the forward part of your feet on top of the book. Rest your heels on the floor. Lift up; lower heels to floor. Do this 10 times.

Sit down for these exercises:

3. Put a pencil on the floor in front of you and pick up the pencil 3 times, grasping it with the curled toes of each foot.

4. Extend your legs out in front of you. Point your right foot forward as you flex your left foot back. Alternate feet. Point each foot 10 times.

Eleven o'clock exercise break: mat exercises to relax you and tone your muscles.

Seated extended stretch

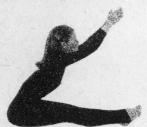

1. Sit with legs together straight out in front of you. Lift arms to meet above head, palms together.

2. Bend down keeping spine straight, arms extended, and legs flat on floor.

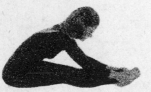

3. Grasp ankles with hands and hold for a count of 5. Return to starting position. Repeat 5 times.

Crisscross

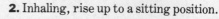

1. Lie on your back, hands clasped behind your head. Have knees bent and feet flat on floor.

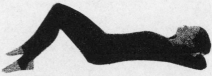

2. Inhaling, rise up to a sitting position.

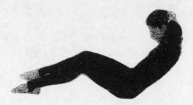
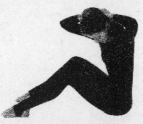

3. Touch right elbow to left knee. Exhaling, slowly lie down.

4. Repeat, touching left elbow to right knee. Alternate 10 times.

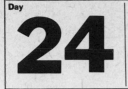 24 | Wednesday

---

Morning

On arising: **breathing exercise.** Stand by the side of your bed with feet together, spine erect, and shoulders relaxed. Begin by exhaling completely. Take in a deep breath through the nostrils. Try to fill your lungs to capacity. Hold breath for a moment. Exhale slowly and steadily, making a humming sound as you do so. Empty lungs completely. Wait a moment and then repeat exercise. Do 10 inhalations and exhalations.

After breathing exercises: **wake-up exercises.**

Waist stretch

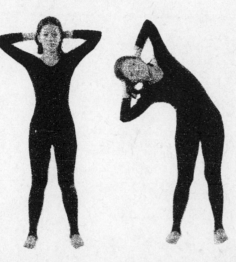

1. Stand with feet shoulder width apart. Clasp hands behind head and lift up rib cage.

2. Bend to the right side, back to center, and then to the left. Repeat 10 times.

Running in place. Always run on a carpeted or padded surface. Warm up by jogging very slowly for 50 steps. Rest for a moment and then run at a faster pace for 4 minutes. Cool down by walking around, taking long strides, until your pulse rate and breathing have returned to normal.

Weigh yourself and record your weight.

Breakfast menu (240 calories)

1 4-ounce glass orange juice (55 calories)
¾ cup bran flakes (101 calories)
½ cup blueberries (40 calories)
1 4-ounce glass skim milk (44 calories)
Coffee (regular or decaffeinated) or tea (no sugar)

Brown-bag lunch: If you are taking lunch to your office, prepare it right after breakfast.

Note: Transfer 4-ounce hamburger patty (from Day 14) from freezer to refrigerator.

"Praise is the best diet for us, after all."
—REVEREND SIDNEY SMITH (1771–1845)

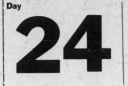

Wednesday

Daytime

Midmorning break: **herb tea.**

Lunch menu (224 calories)
*Vegetable and cottage cheese salad (160 calories)
3 melba toast rounds (24 calories)
½ apple (40 calories)
Coffee (regular or decaffeinated) or tea (no sugar or milk)

*Vegetable and cottage cheese salad
½ cup cottage cheese (120 calories)
1 carrot, chopped (17 calories)
4 radishes, chopped (7 calories)
1 scallion, thinly sliced (4 calories)

1 teaspoon parsley, chopped
2 romaine lettuce leaves (5 calories)
1 tablespoon low-calorie Italian salad
    dressing (7 calories)

Put cottage cheese on lettuce leaves. Sprinkle vegetables over the top. Drizzle dressing over all immediately before serving.

Midafternoon break: Do the spine stretch. Run in place for 1 minute. Relax with a cup of herb tea.

Evening

Dinner menu (535 calories)
*1 broiled hamburger, 4 ounces (252 calories)
1 hamburger bun, toasted (110 calories)
1 slice onion (5 calories)
*1 baked tomato (49 calories)
Tossed green salad made from 2 cups Boston and romaine lettuce leaves,
   torn into bite-sized pieces (15 calories) and 4 sliced radishes (7 calories);
   serve with 1 tablespoon low-calorie bleu-cheese dressing (12 calories)
1 pear (95 calories)
Coffee (regular or decaffeinated) or tea (no sugar or milk)

*Broiled hamburger

¼ pound ground round steak   Pinch of salt
   (252 calories)   Sprinkle of pepper

Combine ingredients and shape into patty. Broil 4 inches from flame for 4 to 5 minutes on each side. Toast hamburger bun under broiler for the last few minutes of cooking time. Serve hamburger on bun, with onion slice.

*Baked tomato

1 tomato (44 calories)   2 teaspoons parsley, chopped (2 calories)
2 teaspoons onion, chopped (3 calories)   ¼ teaspoon oregano

Cut tomato in half and place in small baking pan. Combine onion, parsley, and oregano. Sprinkle over both halves. Bake in oven while hamburger is broiling.

Eleven o'clock exercise break: mat exercises to relax you and tone your muscles.

Pelvic press

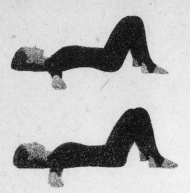

Lie on your back, knees bent and arms at sides. Contract stomach muscles so that spine flattens against floor. Hold for a count of 5 and then release. Repeat 10 times.

Knee lift

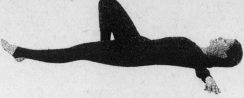

1. Lie on your back, arms extended at shoulder level.

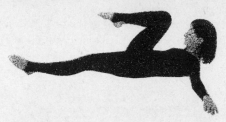

2. Bring left knee up and, at the same time, lift head so that forehead reaches toward knee.

3. Repeat with right knee. Alternate knees, bringing each knee up 10 times.

Last thing before going to bed: **relaxation technique.** Read exercise all the way through before you start.

Lie on your back on a mat, with legs slightly separated and relaxed, arms at your sides, palms of hands facing up. Lift your right leg and shake it vigorously. Let it drop to the mat. Do the same with your left leg. Then shake your right arm and let it drop to the mat. Do the same with your left arm. Lie quietly, breathing in and out deeply 3 times. Lift your hands and clasp your neck. Massage the back of your neck gently and thoroughly and then massage behind your ears. Return arms to sides and inhale and exhale deeply 3 times.

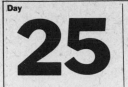

Morning

On arising: **breathing exercise.** Stand by the side of your bed with feet together, spine erect, and shoulders relaxed. Begin by exhaling completely. Take in a deep breath through the nostrils. Try to fill your lungs to capacity. Hold breath for a moment. Exhale slowly and steadily, making a humming sound as you do so. Empty lungs completely. Wait a moment and then repeat exercise. Do 10 inhalations and exhalations.

After breathing exercises: **wake-up exercises.**

Arm and leg stretch

1. Stand with feet together, arms down at sides. Stretch right arm up and forward and left leg back, pointing toes. Stretch fully without straining. Hold position for a count of 5.

2. Repeat, lifting left arm up and extending right leg back. Alternate 10 times to a side.

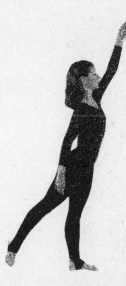

Running in place. Always run on a carpeted or padded surface. Warm up by jogging very slowly for 50 steps. Rest for a moment and then run at a faster pace, lifting feet 4 inches from the floor. Run for 4 minutes. Cool down by walking around, taking long strides, until your pulse rate and breathing have returned to normal.

Weigh yourself and record your weight.

Breakfast menu (245 calories)
1 4-ounce glass orange juice (55 calories)
1 egg, scrambled in nonstick pan (78 calories)
1 slice whole wheat toast (68 calories)
1 4-ounce glass skim milk (44 calories)
Coffee (regular or decaffeinated) or tea (no sugar)

Brown-bag lunch: If you are taking lunch to your office, prepare it right after breakfast.

"Step after step the ladder is ascended."
—HERBERT

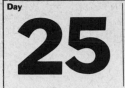

Daytime

Midmorning break: **herb tea.**

Lunch menu (279 calories)
*Vegetarian chef's salad (165 calories)
3 melba toast rounds (24 calories)
1 apple (90 calories)
Coffee (regular or decaffeinated) or tea (no sugar or milk)

***Vegetarian chef's salad**

1 1-ounce slice Swiss cheese, cut into thin strips (106 calories)
4 cherry tomatoes, halved (16 calories)
1 scallion, thinly sliced (4 calories)
1 carrot, pared into curls (17 calories)

¼ head romaine lettuce, torn into bite-sized pieces (10 calories)
1 tablespoon low-calorie bleu-cheese salad dressing (12 calories)

Combine ingredients and toss with dressing immediately before serving.

Midafternoon break: Stand erect. Stretch arms up over head. Lower arms and shake shoulders. Run in place for 1 minute. Relax after cooling off with a cup of herb tea.

Evening

Dinner menu (425 calories)
*Ginger-broiled shrimp (125 calories)
½ cup cooked white rice (112 calories)
¼ pound spinach, steamed (22 calories) and sprinkled with 1 teaspoon soy
    sauce (2 calories) mixed with 2 teaspoons lemon juice (2 calories) and 1
    tablespoon sesame seeds (55 calories)
1 banana, sliced (80 calories) in ¼ cup fresh orange juice (27 calories)
Coffee (regular or decaffeinated) or tea (no sugar or milk)

*Ginger-broiled shrimp

10 shrimp (100 calories)
1 tablespoon soy sauce (10 calories)
1 teaspoon safflower oil (40 calories)

½ clove garlic, pressed in garlic press
    (1 calorie)
1 teaspoon grated fresh ginger or ½
    teaspoon ground ginger

Clean and devein shrimp. In a glass or ceramic bowl combine soy sauce, safflower oil, garlic, and ginger. Add shrimp to mixture and marinate for at least ½ hour. Thread shrimp onto small skewers and broil 4 inches from heat for 3 to 4 minutes on each side.

Beauty break: **how to have beautiful, healthy feet—part 2.** For some mysterious reason, a great many people either ignore or mistreat their feet, as though they were not worthy objects of concern. But like most other things in life, feet respond well to tender loving care. When you start taking good care of your feet and wearing properly fitted shoes, you will find such an improvement in your physical well-being that you may even feel like dancing. And as everybody knows, dancing is great for both your body and your spirits. Beside massage and exercise, the best way to keep your feet in shape is to make a leisurely pedicure a regular twice-a-month part of your beauty and health program. Here's how to give yourself a pedicure that will keep your feet looking and feeling terrific. (The list of equipment seems long, but most of the items are very inexpensive and will last a long time.)

You will need: nail polish remover, cotton pads, basin of warm soapy water, toenail clippers, pumice stone, emery board, cuticle remover, orangewood stick, facial tissues, and polish (plus base coat if you use it).

    If you have been wearing polish on your toenails, remove it. Soak feet and pumice stone in warm soapy water for 5 minutes. (While feet are soaking, flex and point toes to stretch and tone the muscles.) After 5 minutes, use the pumice stone to rub away any rough or calloused skin. Using a moderate amount of pressure and a circular motion, go over every rough spot on your feet. Don't forget your heels. Rinse feet with cool water and dry with a towel. Clip nails with clippers, cutting straight across. Use an emery board to smooth any rough spots. Do not file into the corners of your nails because this practice can lead to ingrown toenails. Dip a cotton-wrapped orangewood stick into cuticle remover and apply liberally around the edges of the nail and under nail tips. Wait 3 minutes and then use the wrapped orangewood stick to push the cuticles gently back. Rinse feet in warm water and dry thoroughly. If you are going to apply polish, use 2-inch lengths of twisted tissue between toes to separate them. Apply base coat, let dry for 5 minutes, and then apply two coats of polish, letting the first coat dry well before you apply the next. If you are uncertain about what color to use on toenails, try one of the new neutrals—sand-biege, mauve, or nude.

Eleven o'clock exercise break: mat exercises to relax you and tone your muscles.

Seated body twist

1. Sit with legs wide apart. Lift arms straight up, palms turned inward.

2. Slowly twist body to face right foot.

3. Bend down, keeping arms beside head and bringing head as close to leg as possible.

4. Return to starting position and stretch to the left. Repeat 5 times to each side.

Morning

On arising: **breathing exercise.** Stand by the side of your bed with feet together, spine erect, and shoulders relaxed. Begin by exhaling completely. Take in a deep breath through the nostrils. Try to fill your lungs to capacity. Hold breath for a moment. Exhale slowly and steadily, making a humming sound as you do so. Empty lungs completely. Wait a moment and then repeat exercise. Do 10 inhalations and exhalations.

After breathing exercises: **wake-up exercises.**

Clasped hand stretch

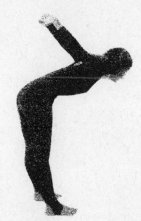

1. Stand with feet 3 inches apart. Link fingers behind back.

2. Lean forward from the hips and lift arms.

3. Lean as far forward as comfortable. Straighten up and return to starting position. Repeat 10 times.

Running in place. Always run on a carpeted or padded surface. Warm up by jogging very slowly for 50 steps. Rest for a moment and then run at a faster pace, lifting feet 4 inches from the floor. Run for 4 minutes. Cool down by walking around, taking long strides, until your pulse rate and breathing have returned to normal.

Weigh yourself and record your weight.

Breakfast menu (237 calories)
1 4-ounce glass orange juice (55 calories)
¼ cup pineapple cottage cheese, to use as spread on toast (70 calories)
1 slice whole wheat toast (68 calories)
1 4-ounce glass skim milk (44 calories)
Coffee (regular or decaffeinated) or tea (no sugar)

Brown-bag lunch: If you are taking lunch to your office, prepare it right after breakfast.

Note: Transfer ground lamb from freezer to refrigerator.

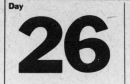

Day 26 | # Friday

Daytime

Midmorning break: **herb tea.**

Lunch menu (253 calories)
*Open-faced shrimp salad sandwich (197 calories)
1 carrot, cut into sticks (17 calories)
1 tangerine (39 calories)
Coffee (regular or decaffeinated) or tea (no sugar or milk)

*Open-faced shrimp salad sandwich

8 boiled shrimp, chopped (80 calories)
1 scallion, thinly sliced (4 calories)
1 stalk celery, chopped (5 calories)

1 tablespoon diet or imitation
  mayonnaise (48 calories)
2 leaves romaine lettuce (5 calories)
½ hamburger bun (55 calories)

Combine shrimp, scallion, celery, and mayonnaise. Put lettuce leaves on bun and top with shrimp mixture.

Midafternoon break: Run in place for 1 minute. After cooling off, drink a cup of herb tea.

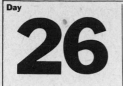

Friday

Evening

Dinner menu (518 calories)

1 8-ounce glass mineral water with ice and a thin slice of lemon

*2 Armenian ground-lamb kebabs (373 calories)

2 carrots, sliced and boiled (34 calories) and sprinkled with 1 teaspoon lemon juice and grated lemon peel (1 calorie)

1 zucchini, sliced, boiled, and sprinkled with pinch marjoram (26 calories)

Tossed green salad made from 2 cups Boston and romaine lettuce leaves, torn into bite-sized pieces (15 calories), ½ cucumber, peeled and cubed (10 calories), and 4 sliced radishes (7 calories); serve with 1 tablespoon low-calorie Italian salad dressing (7 calories)

½ cup canned apricots, water-packed (45 calories)

Coffee (regular or decaffeinated) or tea (no sugar or milk)

*Armenian ground-lamb kebabs

½ pound ground lamb (736 calories)
½ teaspoon salt
¼ teaspoon black pepper
¼ teaspoon ground cumin

¼ teaspoon ground coriander
¼ teaspoon oregano
2 scallions, thinly sliced (8 calories)
1 tablespoon parsley, chopped (2 calories)

In a mixing bowl combine lamb, salt, pepper, cumin, coriander, oregano, and 1 scallion. Mix the ingredients thoroughly, using your hands or a large spoon. Form the mixture into 4 sausage-shaped rolls. Push 6-inch skewers through the centers of the rolls. Broil 4 inches from heat until done, turning to brown on all sides, about 10 minutes in all. Serve 2 rolls sprinkled with chopped parsley and scallion. Freeze remaining 2, when cool, for later use.

Eleven o'clock exercise break: mat exercises to relax you and tone your muscles.

Kneeling leg lift

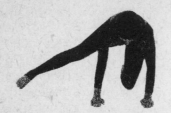

1. Kneel with hands and feet flat on floor.

2. Move right leg out to side at a right angle to your body.

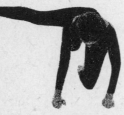

3. Lift foot up. Hold for a count of 5 and return to starting position.

4. Repeat with left leg. Alternate legs 3 times.

Roll ups

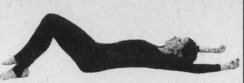

1. Lie on your back, arms extended above your head. Have knees bent and feet flat on floor.

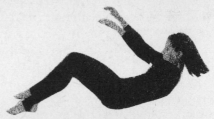

2. Inhaling, slowly rise up to a sitting position.

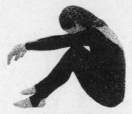

3. Stretch forward with your arms, touching your feet or shins. Exhaling, slowly return to starting position. Repeat 10 times.

Last thing before you go to bed: **relaxation technique.** Read through the exercise before you start.

Lie flat on your back on a mat. Legs should be relaxed. Arms are close to your sides, palms of hands facing up. Close your eyes and take two deep breaths. With your mind's eye, you are going to touch each part of your body and relax it. Start with your toes. Imagine you can touch your big toe with your mind; relax it. Move from toe to toe on the right foot. Then, as though your mind had a kind of relaxing ray, move up to the right ankle, the shin, the knee, the thigh. Now do your left foot and leg. Slowly cover the entire body, including the top of the head, the ears, the back of the head, the nape of the neck, and the spine, always focusing the beam of your mind on each part of your body to relax it. When you have finished, lie quietly for a few minutes and concentrate on your deep breathing.

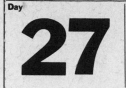

Morning

On arising: **breathing exercise.** Stand by the side of your bed with feet together, spine erect, and shoulders relaxed. Begin by exhaling completely. Take in a deep breath through the nostrils. Try to fill your lungs to capacity. Hold breath for a moment. Exhale slowly and steadily, making a humming sound as you do so. Empty lungs completely. Wait a moment and then repeat exercise. Do 10 inhalations and exhalations.

After breathing exercises: **wake-up exercises.**

Waist stretch

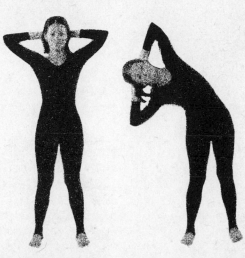

1. Stand with feet shoulder width apart. Clasp hands behind head and lift up rib cage.

2. Bend to the right side, back to center, and then to the left. Repeat 10 times.

Running in place. Always run on a carpeted or padded surface. Warm up by jogging very slowly for 50 steps. Rest for a moment and then run at a faster pace for 4½ minutes. Cool down by walking around, taking long strides, until your pulse rate and breathing have returned to normal.

Weigh yourself and record your weight.

Breakfast menu (289 calories)

½ grapefruit (48 calories)

*3 cottage cheese pancakes (142 calories)

½ cup unsweetened applesauce, mixed with ½ teaspoon cinnamon (55 calories)

1 4-ounce glass skim milk (44 calories)

Coffee (regular or decaffeinated) or tea (no sugar)

*Cottage cheese pancakes

½ cup cottage cheese (120 calories)

1 egg (78 calories)

1 tablespoon flour (28 calories)

2 teaspoons wheat germ (18 calories)

1 teaspoon safflower oil (40 calories)

¼ teaspoon vanilla

Combine all ingredients in a mixing bowl and stir to blend thoroughly. Heat nonstick frying pan over medium heat. Drop 3 tablespoons of batter into hot pan. Cook for about 3 minutes until brown, then turn with a spatula to brown the other side. Serve topped with cinnamon applesauce. Makes 6 pancakes. Reserve remaining batter for breakfast on Day 29.

Shopping List

Dairy products

1 8-ounce container plain yogurt

1 quart skim milk

Fruits and vegetables

1 2½-inch apple

1 7-inch banana

½ pound seedless green grapes

1 4-inch grapefruit

3 3-inch oranges

3 lemons

1 bunch broccoli

½ pound medium mushrooms (about 16)

1 5-inch yellow summer squash

1 pound potatoes (3 to a pound)

1 bunch parsley

1 bunch scallions

1 head romaine lettuce

2 7-inch cucumbers

2 3-inch tomatoes

1 8-ounce can tomato sauce

½ pound spinach

1 head Boston lettuce

1 head iceberg lettuce

1 8¼-ounce can whole tomatoes

Meat and fish

½ pound veal stew meat (shoulder)

¼ pound ground beef round

2 12-ounce chicken breasts

1 3½-ounce can solid white tuna, water-packed

1 4-ounce filet mignon (store in freezer)

Other items

1 6-ounce box egg noodles

1 11-ounce bottle mineral water

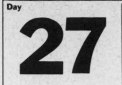

Daytime

Lunch menu (228 calories)
*Grilled cheese and tomato sandwich (171 calories)
4 radishes (7 calories)
½ cup green grapes (50 calories)
Coffee (regular or decaffeinated) or tea (no sugar or milk)

*Grilled cheese and tomato sandwich

1 1-ounce slice Swiss cheese (106 calories)	Pinch of oregano
2 slices tomato (10 calories)	½ hamburger bun (55 calories)

Lightly toast the bun. Place tomato slices on bun and sprinkle with oregano. Put cheese slice on top and broil until cheese melts.

Midafternoon break: Run in place for 1 minute.

Beauty break: **choosing a new fragrance.** Many delightful new fragrances have been created in the past few years—light floral combinations, green woodsy scents, and musky Oriental blends. With so many exciting fragrances to choose from, it can be a pleasure to wear a different one for different moods and occasions. Yet a great many women fall into the habit of wearing only one scent. Sometimes it's only when a friend wears a new fragrance that we are tempted to experiment. Try a new fragrance on your own. Use the testers provided by perfume companies—department, drug, and discount stores usually have them. Try just two scents at a time with a dab on each wrist. Wait about half an hour for the oils to be absorbed into the skin, then whiff. Another day try two more, and you'll eventually have a few mood-uplifting perfumes suited just to you.

Beauty break checklist for upcoming week
36 small hair rollers or rods
pH-balanced protein shampoo
Hair dryer
Widetoothed comb

2

Evening

Dinner menu (526 calories)

*Baked Tandoori chicken (205 calories)

1 yellow summer squash, sliced, steamed, and sprinkled with 1 teaspoon chopped parsley (40 calories)

*Chopped vegetable salad (61 calories)

1 breadstick (40 calories)

½ banana, sliced (40 calories) and topped with ½ cup vanilla yogurt (100 calories) and 1 tablespoon chopped walnuts (40 calories)

Coffee (regular or decaffeinated) or tea (no sugar or milk)

*Baked Tandoori chicken

1 12-ounce chicken breast, skinned and cut in half (288 calories)

1 onion, chopped (38 calories)

1 clove garlic (3 calories)

1 small slice fresh ginger or ½ teaspoon ground ginger (2 calories)

1 tablespoon lemon juice (3 calories)

½ cup plain yogurt (75 calories)

½ teaspoon ground coriander

½ teaspoon ground cumin

½ teaspoon salt

Black pepper to taste

½ teaspoon paprika

Put onion, garlic, ginger, and lemon juice in blender and blend until smooth. Transfer mixture to a large bowl. Add yogurt, coriander, cumin, salt, and pepper. Stir to blend thoroughly. Put chicken breasts in yogurt marinade, coating thoroughly. Let chicken marinate for 3 to 4 hours, turning several times. Remove from marinade and put in small baking dish. Bake in a 350° oven for 45 minutes. Sprinkle with paprika. Brown under broiler flame for 2 minutes or so. Serve ½ tonight; reserve ½ for lunch on Day 30.

*Chopped vegetable salad

1 tomato, chopped (44 calories)

½ cucumber, peeled and chopped (10 calories)

1 scallion, thinly sliced (4 calories)

1 tablespoon lemon juice (3 calories)

¼ teaspoon cumin

Salt and pepper

Combine all ingredients and mix thoroughly.

Eleven o'clock exercise break: mat exercises to relax you and tone your muscles.

Side leg lifts

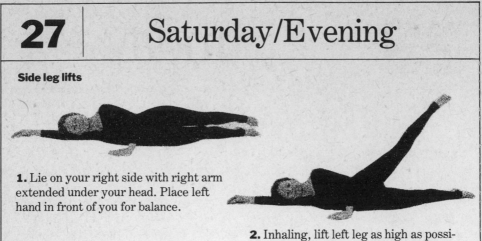

1. Lie on your right side with right arm extended under your head. Place left hand in front of you for balance.

2. Inhaling, lift left leg as high as possible. Exhaling, slowly lower leg. Repeat 10 times with each leg.

Pelvic press

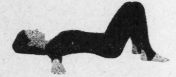 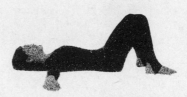

Lie on your back, knees bent and arms at sides. Contract stomach muscles so that spine flattens against floor. Hold for a count of 5 and then release. Repeat 10 times.

Sunday

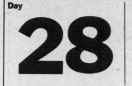

Morning

On arising: **breathing exercise.** Stand by the side of the bed with feet together, spine erect, and shoulders relaxed. Begin by exhaling completely. Take in a deep breath through the nostrils. Try to fill your lungs to capacity. Hold breath for a moment. Exhale slowly and steadily, making a humming sound as you do so. Empty lungs completely. Wait a moment and then repeat exercise. Do 10 inhalations and exhalations.

Immediately after breathing exercise: **wake-up exercises.**

Shoulder stretch

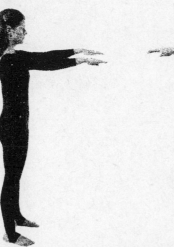 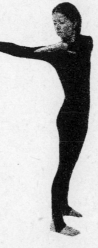

1. Stand with feet shoulder width apart. Raise arms to shoulder height and straight out in front of you.

2. Twist at waist and swing both arms back to the right without straining and then swing them to the left. Repeat 10 times to each side.

Weigh yourself and record your weight.

Breakfast menu (266 calories)
½ grapefruit (48 calories)
*Parsley-cheese omelet (106 calories)
1 slice whole wheat toast (68 calories)
1 4-ounce glass skim milk (44 calories)
Coffee (regular or decaffeinated) or tea (no sugar)

*Parsley-cheese omelet

1 egg (78 calories)
1 teaspoon cold water
1 tablespoon Swiss cheese, grated or

finely chopped (26 calories)
1 tablespoon parsley, chopped
(2 calories)

Add water to egg and beat just enough to mix. Heat nonstick frying pan over high heat. Pour in egg and tilt to spread evenly over the surface of the pan. When egg is nearly cooked, sprinkle with cheese and parsley. With a spatula, gently fold omelet over. Slide onto warmed plate.

Exercise break: **nature walk.** Go for a brisk 3-mile walk in a specially beautiful part of your city or town. Go with a friend and share the pleasure.

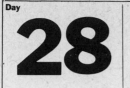

Sunday

Daytime

Lunch menu (239 calories)
*Open-faced tuna salad sandwich (214 calories)
¼ cup green grapes (25 calories)
Coffee (regular or decaffeinated) or tea (no sugar or milk)

*Open-faced tuna salad sandwich

1 3½-ounce can solid white tuna,
   water-packed (120 calories)
1 teaspoon capers (3 calories)
1 tablespoon parsley, chopped
   (2 calories)

2 teaspoons imitation or diet mayonnaise
   (32 calories)
1 leaf romaine lettuce (2 calories)
½ hamburger bun (55 calories)

Combine drained tuna, capers, parsley, and mayonnaise and mix thoroughly. Tear romaine lettuce leaf into small pieces. Cover bun with lettuce, then with tuna salad.

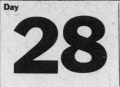

Sunday

Evening

Dinner menu (515 calories)
1 11-ounce glass mineral water with ice and a thin slice of lime
*Veal stew Marengo (311 calories)
1 potato, boiled in jacket (90 calories)
Tossed green salad made with 2 cups Boston and romaine lettuce leaves, torn into bite-sized pieces (15 calories) and sprinkled with 1 tablespoon chopped parsley (2 calories); serve with 1 tablespoon low-calorie Italian salad dressing (7 calories)
*½ apple and orange fruit cup (90 calories)
Coffee (regular or decaffeinated) or tea (no sugar or milk)

*Veal stew Marengo
½ pound veal stew meat (shoulder), cut into 1-inch cubes (494 calories)
¼ teaspoon thyme
¼ teaspoon basil
1 onion, peeled and chopped (38 calories)
1 bay leaf
1 clove garlic, minced (3 calories)
6 mushrooms, sliced (30 calories)
1 8¼-ounce can whole tomatoes (50 calories)
1 tablespoon parsley, chopped (2 calories)
1 cup chicken broth, made from bouillon cube (5 calories)

Brown veal in a nonstick frying pan, turning to sear evenly. Add onion, garlic, and tomatoes and simmer for 3 minutes. Transfer to a flameproof casserole and add chicken broth, thyme, basil, and bay leaf. Simmer for 1 hour. Add sliced mushrooms and simmer for 10 minutes more. Sprinkle with chopped parsley. Serve ½ of the stew tonight; reserve ½ for dinner on Day 30.

*Apple and orange fruit cup
1 apple, cored and cut into cubes (90 calories)
1 orange, peeled and cut into cubes (64 calories)
¼ cup orange juice (27 calories)
Mix all together. Serve ½ recipe tonight; reserve remainder for dinner on Day 29.

Eleven o'clock exercise break: mat exercises to relax you and tone your muscles.

Side leg lifts

1. Lie on your right side with right arm extended under your head. Place left hand in front of you for balance.

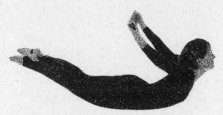

2. Inhaling, lift left leg as high as possible. Exhaling, slowly lower leg. Repeat 10 times with each leg.

Body curl up

1. Lie on your stomach, legs together. Put arms behind back, holding one end of a hand towel in each hand.

2. Slowly raise head, feet, and hands. Pulling towel taut, hold for a count of 3. Repeat 5 times.

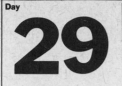
Monday

Morning

On arising: **breathing exercise.** Stand by the side of the bed with feet together, spine erect, and shoulders relaxed. Begin by exhaling completely. You should be able to hear the exhalation. Next, inhale slowly and deeply through your nostrils. Your mouth should be closed. As you breathe in, lift your rib cage and contract your abdominal muscles. Fill lungs to capacity. Hold breath for a moment. Then exhale slowly and steadily until you feel you have completely emptied your lungs. Keep abdominal muscles contracted. Again, wait for a moment; then inhale and repeat the exercise. Do this 10 times.

Immediately after breathing exercise: **wake-up exercises.**

Backward arm swing

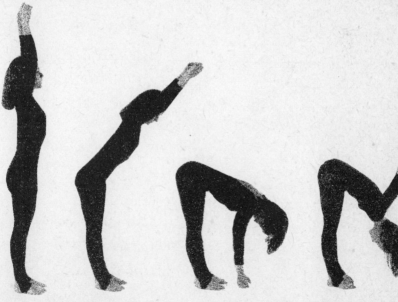

1. Stand with feet together. Raise arms straight up, palms turned in.

2. Bend forward as far as you can, swinging arms down and back behind you as far as is comfortable.

3. Swing back to starting position, keeping shoulders relaxed throughout. Do 5 slow swings and 5 fast ones.

Running in place. Always run on a carpeted or padded surface. Warm up by jogging very slowly for 50 steps. Rest for a moment and then run at a faster pace for 5 minutes. Cool down by walking around, taking long strides, until your pulse rate and breathing have returned to normal.

Weigh yourself and record your weight.

Breakfast menu (268 calories)
1 4-ounce glass orange juice (55 calories)
3 cottage cheese pancakes (from Day 27) (142 calories)
¼ cup unsweetened applesauce, mixed with ¼ teaspoon cinnamon (27 calories)
1 4-ounce glass skim milk (44 calories)
Coffee (regular or decaffeinated) or tea (no sugar)

Brown-bag lunch: If you are taking lunch to your office, prepare it right after breakfast.

"Do not turn back when you are just at the goal."
—PUBLIUS SYRUS

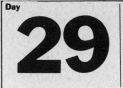

Monday

Daytime

Midmorning break: **herb tea.**

Lunch menu (246 calories)
*Open-faced Swiss cheese sandwich (221 calories)
¼ cup green grapes (25 calories)
Coffee (regular or decaffeinated) or tea (no sugar or milk)

*Open-faced Swiss cheese sandwich

1 1-ounce slice Swiss cheese (106 calories)
2 slices tomato (10 calories)
1 leaf romaine lettuce (2 calories)

1 tablespoon diet mayonnaise (48 calories)
½ hamburger bun (55 calories)
Pinch of marjoram

Lightly toast bun and spread on mayonnaise. Put romaine lettuce leaf on bun, then tomato slices. Sprinkle with marjoram. Place cheese on top and melt under broiler.

Midafternoon break: Stand erect and shake arms and hands vigorously. Shake each leg vigorously. Run in place for 1 minute. After cooling off, relax with cold mineral water with a thin slice of lemon.

Evening

Dinner menu (494 calories)
*Broiled Oriental hamburger (259 calories)
1 potato, peeled, boiled in lightly salted water (90 calories), and sprinkled
   with 1 tablespoon chopped parsley (2 calories)
Tossed green salad made with ¼ pound fresh spinach, torn into bite-sized
   pieces (22 calories), 4 sliced radishes (7 calories), and 1 carrot, shaved into
   curls (17 calories); serve with 1 tablespoon low-calorie Italian salad
   dressing (7 calories)
½ apple and orange fruit cup (from Day 28) (90 calories)
Coffee (regular or decaffeinated) or tea (no sugar or milk)

Broiled Oriental hamburger
¼ pound ground beef round   1 scallion, thinly sliced (4 calories)
   (252 calories)   Pinch ground ginger
1 teaspoon soy sauce (3 calories)

Combine all ingredients in a bowl and mix thoroughly. Shape meat into patty. Broil 4 inches from flame, 4 to 5 minutes on each side, or to desired degree of doneness.

Eleven o'clock exercise break: mat exercises to relax you and tone your muscles.

Body curl up

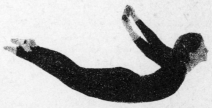

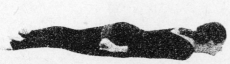

1. Lie on your stomach, legs together. Put arms behind back, holding one end of a hand towel in each hand.

2. Slowly raise head, feet, and hands. Pulling towel taut, hold for a count of 3. Repeat 5 times.

Seated body twist

1. Sit with legs wide apart. Lift arms straight up, palms turned inward.

2. Slowly twist body to face right foot.

3. Bend down, keeping arms beside head and bringing head as close to leg as possible.

4. Return to starting position and stretch to the left. Repeat 5 times to each side.

Last thing before you go to bed: **relaxation technique.** Read exercise all the way through before you do it.

Lie on your back on a mat, with legs slightly separated and relaxed, arms at your sides, palms of hands facing up. Lift your right leg and shake it vigorously. Let it drop to the mat. Do the same with your left leg. Then shake your right arm and let it drop to the mat. Do the same with your left arm. Lie quietly, breathing in and out deeply 3 times. Lift your hands and clasp your neck. Massage the back of your neck gently and thoroughly and then massage behind your ears. Return arms to sides and inhale deeply 3 times.

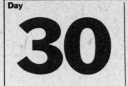

Morning

On arising: **breathing exercise.** Stand by the side of the bed with feet together, spine erect, and shoulder relaxed. Begin the exercise by exhaling completely. You should be able to hear the exhalation. Next, inhale slowly and deeply through your nostrils. Your mouth should be closed. As you breathe in, lift your rib cage and contract your abdominal muscles. Fill lungs to capacity. Hold breath for a moment. Then exhale slowly and steadily until you feel you have completely emptied your lungs. Keep abdominal muscles contracted. Again, wait for a moment, then inhale and repeat the exercise. Do this 10 times.

Immediately after breathing exercise: **wake-up exercises.**

Fencer's lunge

1. Stand with feet 2½ feet apart. Raise arms to shoulder height. Bend right knee and shift weight to the right. Hold for a count of 5 and return to center.

2. Bend left knee and shift weight to the left. Hold for a count of 5 and return to center. Repeat 10 times to each side.

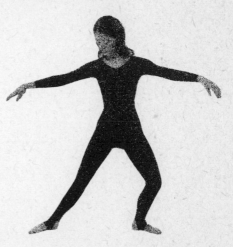

Running in place. Always run on a carpeted or padded surface. Warm up by jogging very slowly for 50 steps. Rest for a moment and then run at a faster pace for 5 minutes. Cool down by walking around, taking long strides, until your pulse rate and breathing have returned to normal.

Weigh yourself and record your weight.

Breakfast menu (240 calories)

1 4-ounce glass orange juice (55 calories)
¾ cup bran flakes (101 calories)
½ banana, sliced on cereal (40 calories)
1 4-ounce glass skim milk (44 calories)
Coffee (regular or decaffeinated) or tea (no sugar)

Brown-bag lunch: If you are taking lunch to your office, prepare it right after breakfast.

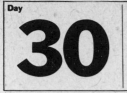

Daytime

Midmorning break: **herb tea.**

Lunch menu (274 calories)
*Chicken and romaine salad (242 calories)
4 melba toast rounds (32 calories)
Coffee (regular or decaffeinated) or tea (no sugar or milk)

*Chicken and romaine salad

½ baked Tandoori chicken breast (from Day 27), sliced into julienne strips (205 calories)
½ cucumber, peeled and cut into strips (10 calories)
1 teaspoon capers (3 calories)

1 scallion, thinly sliced (4 calories)
¼ head romaine lettuce, torn into bite-sized pieces (10 calories)
1 tablespoon low-calorie Italian salad dressing (7 calories)
1 tablespoon lemon juice (3 calories)

Combine ingredients. Toss with salad dressing and lemon juice immediately before serving.

Midafternoon break: Stand erect and take 5 deep breaths. Run in place for 1 minute. After cooling off, drink a cup of herb tea.

Tuesday

Evening

Dinner menu (499 calories)
Veal stew Marengo (reheated from Day 28) (311 calories)
½ cup cooked egg noodles, sprinkled with 1 teaspoon poppy seeds
(100 calories)
2 stalks broccoli, steamed (36 calories) and sprinkled with 2 teaspoons lemon
juice (2 calories)
½ cup green grapes (50 calories)
Coffee (regular or decaffeinated) or tea (no sugar or milk)

Beauty break: **a curly hair style.** Curly hair is appealing and easy to wear. If you have been thinking about getting a permanent or letting your natural curl have its way, try the curly hair style suggested here (which will work on all but very long hair). If you like the effect and your hair is straight, you may want to get a permanent, or perhaps wear this curly style only occasionally—when you feel like a change.

You will need: 36 small foam-rubber rollers or large permanent-wave rods, pH-balanced protein shampoo, hair dryer, and a wide-toothed comb.

Wash hair thoroughly with protein shampoo. Blot dry with a towel. Use a wide-toothed comb to remove snarls and tangles. Section hair down the center and from ear to ear so that you have four manageable sections to work with. For an all-over curly effect, follow directions exactly. Beginning at the front of the right front section, roll hair from the ends down over the curler—each lock of hair should have about a 1-inch-square base on the scalp. Make neat, even rows of curlers as you move from the front to the back on the right side. Then do the same on the left side. Now dry thoroughly with a hair dryer. Unroll a curl to test from time to time. When hair is completely dry, remove curlers and brush hair up all around head. Brush hair down or back to style. If you prefer hair flat on top, place first rollers at temples.

Eleven o'clock exercise break: mat exercises to relax you and tone your muscles.

Knee bends and squeeze

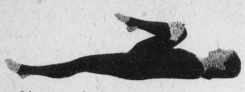

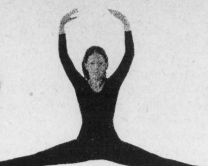

1. Lie on your back, arms at sides and palms up. Inhaling, raise right knee to chest. Clasp knee with hands and hold for a count of 5. Exhaling, lower right leg.

2. Repeat with left knee. Raise each knee 5 times.

1. Sit with legs wide apart. Lift arms straight up, palms turned inward.

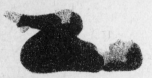

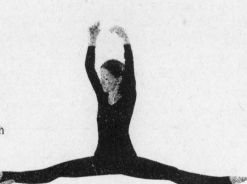

3. Raise both knees together. Clasp with hands and pull in for a count of 5. Straighten legs and lower slowly. Repeat 5 times with both legs.

2. Slowly twist body to face right foot.

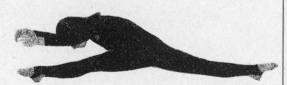

3. Bend down, keeping arms beside head and bringing head as close to leg as possible.

4. Return to starting position and stretch to the left. Repeat 5 times to each side.

Morning

On arising: **breathing exercise.** Stand by the side of the bed with feet together, spine erect, and shoulders relaxed. Begin the exercise by exhaling completely. You should be able to hear the exhalation. Next, inhale slowly and deeply through your nostrils. Your mouth should be closed. As you breathe in, lift your rib cage and contract your abdominal muscles. Fill lungs to capacity. Hold your breath for a moment. Then exhale slowly and steadily until you feel you have completely emptied your lungs. Keep abdominal muscles contracted. Again, wait for a moment, then inhale and repeat the exercise. Do this 10 times.

Immediately after breathing exercise: **wake-up exercises.**

Full extension twist

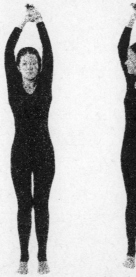

1. Stand with feet together, arms at sides. Breathing in, rise up on toes, lifting arms, linking fingers, and turning up palms.

2. Slowly twist body to right as far as is comfortable. Return to center, lower heels to floor.

3. Repeat, twisting to the left. Twist 5 times to each side.

Running in place. Always run on a carpeted or padded surface. Warm up by jogging very slowly for 50 steps. Rest for a moment and then run at a faster pace for 5 minutes. Cool down by walking around, taking long strides, until your pulse rate and breathing have returned to normal.

Weigh yourself and record your weight. If you are near your ideal weight but not close enough, increase your activity.

Breakfast menu (245 calories)
1 4-ounce glass orange juice (55 calories)
1 egg, scrambled in nonstick pan (78 calories)
1 slice whole wheat toast (68 calories)
1 4-ounce glass skim milk (44 calories)
Coffee (regular or decaffeinated) or tea (no sugar)

Brown-bag lunch: If you are taking lunch to your office, prepare it right after breakfast.

"With ordinary talent and extraordinary perseverance
all things are attainable."
—THOMAS FOWELL BUXTON

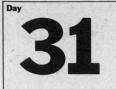

Daytime

Midmorning break: **herb tea.**

Lunch menu (180 calories)
*Open-faced ham sandwich (184 calories)
1 carrot, pared into curls (17 calories)
½ orange (save a piece of rind for afternoon herb tea) (32 calories)
Coffee (regular or decaffeinated) or tea (no sugar or milk)

*Open-faced ham sandwich

1 1-ounce slice boiled ham (53 calories)   1 teaspoon prepared mustard (8 calories)
1 leaf romaine lettuce (2 calories)   1 slice whole wheat bread (68 calories)

Lightly toast the bread and spread on mustard. Top with lettuce leaf and ham.

Midafternoon break: Run in place for 1 minute. Have a cup of herb tea with orange rind.

Evening

Dinner menu (538 calories)
*Chinese chicken with mushrooms and green pepper (287 calories)
½ cup cooked white rice (112 calories)
*Cucumber salad (72 calories)
½ orange, peeled, cut into sections (32 calories) and mixed with ¼ cup
  unsweetened pineapple chunks, packed in own juice (35 calories)
Coffee (regular or decaffeinated) or tea (no sugar or milk)

*Chinese chicken with mushrooms and green pepper

1 12-ounce chicken breast, cut in half (288 calories)	2 scallions, cut into 1-inch lengths (8 calories)
2 teaspoons safflower oil (80 calories)	1 tablespoon soy sauce (10 calories)
½ green pepper, cut into strips (8 calories)	⅓ cup chicken broth, made from bouillon cube (2 calories)
5 mushrooms, sliced (25 calories)	1 teaspoon cornstarch (10 calories)

Remove skin from chicken breast, reserve ½ for following recipe, and slice meat into thin slivers. Heat oil in a nonstick frying pan over high heat. Add chicken and stir to cook, about 2 minutes. Add green pepper, mushrooms, and scallions. Cook for another 2 minutes, stirring to assure even cooking. Combine cornstarch with cooled broth and soy sauce. Stir to mix thoroughly. Add to chicken and vegetables and cook until sauce thickens, about 2 minutes.

Bake remaining half of chicken breast in 350° oven for 45 to 50 minutes. Season with 1 tablespoon lemon juice (3 calories), salt, and pepper. Use for lunch on Day 33.

*Cucumber salad

½ cucumber, peeled and sliced (10 calories)	1 teaspoon soy sauce (3 calories)
1 tablespoon white vinegar (2 calories)	1 teaspoon sugar (17 calories)
1 tablespoon water	1 teaspoon safflower oil (40 calories)

Combine dressing ingredients and mix thoroughly. Pour over cucumber.

Eleven o'clock exercise break: mat exercises to relax you and tone your muscles.

Kneeling leg lift

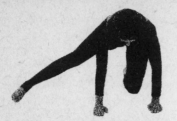

1. Kneel with hands and feet flat on floor.

2. Move right leg out to side at a right angle to your body.

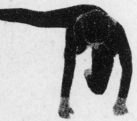

3. Lift foot up. Hold for a count of 5 and return to starting position.

4. Repeat with left leg. Alternate legs 3 times.

Straight leg stretch

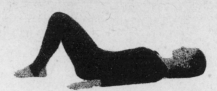

1. Lie on your back, arms at sides and knees bent with feet flat on floor.

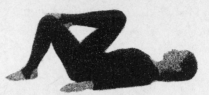

2. Bring right knee to your chest.

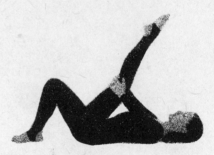

3. Straighten leg and grasp with hands. Pull leg toward you. Release and return to starting position.

4. Repeat with left leg. Alternate, lifting each leg 3 times.

32 | Thursday

Morning

On arising: **breathing exercise.** Stand by the side of the bed with feet together, spine erect, and shoulders relaxed. Begin the exercise by exhaling completely. You should be able to hear the exhalation. Next, inhale slowly and deeply through your nostrils. Your mouth should be closed. As you breathe in, lift your rib cage and contract your abdominal muscles. Fill lungs to capacity. Hold breath for a moment. Then exhale slowly and steadily until you feel you have completely emptied your lungs. Keep abdominal muscles contracted. Again, wait for a moment, then inhale and repeat the exercise. Do this 10 times.

Immediately after breathing exercise: **wake-up exercises.**

Backward arm swing

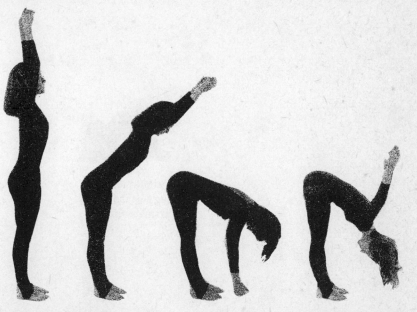

1. Stand with feet together. Raise arms straight up, palms turned in.

2. Bend forward as far as you can, swinging arms down and back behind you as far as is comfortable.

3. Swing back to starting position, keeping shoulders relaxed throughout. Do 5 slow swings and 5 fast ones.

Running in place. Always run on a carpeted or padded surface. Warm up with a slow jog for 50 steps. Arms should be bent at elbows and held close to the body. Lift feet 3 or 4 inches off the floor. Imitate the heel-toe alternation of regular running. After you have warmed up, rest for a moment and then run at a faster pace, lifting legs and feet higher. Run for 5 minutes. Cool down by walking around, taking long strides, until your pulse rate and breathing have returned to normal.

Weigh yourself and record your weight.

Breakfast menu (227 calories)
1 4-ounce glass orange juice (55 calories)
¼ cup cottage cheese, sprinkled with cinnamon, to use as spread on toast (60 calories)
1 slice whole wheat toast (68 calories)
1 4-ounce glass skim milk (44 calories)
Coffee (regular or decaffeinated) or tea (no sugar)

Brown-bag lunch: If you are taking lunch to your office, prepare it right after breakfast.

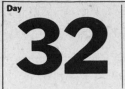

Daytime

Midmorning break: **herb tea.**

Lunch menu (245 calories)
*Spinach salad with hard-cooked egg (181 calories)
3 melba toast rounds (24 calories)
½ banana (40 calories)
Coffee (regular or decaffeinated) or tea (no sugar or milk)

*Spinach salad with hard-cooked egg
½ pound fresh spinach washed, dried, and stems removed (44 calories)
1 egg, hard-cooked and chopped (78 calories)
5 mushrooms, sliced (25 calories)

4 cherry tomatoes (16 calories)
1 scallion, thinly sliced (4 calories)
2 tablespoons low-calorie Italian salad dressing (14 calories)

Prepare egg by placing it in cold water and bringing to a boil. Lower heat and simmer for 6 minutes. Turn off heat and let egg stand for 15 minutes. Remove egg from water and put under cold running water for several minutes. Tear spinach leaves into bite-sized pieces. Combine all ingredients except dressing and toss to mix thoroughly. Add dressing just before eating.

Midafternoon break: Do spine stretch, then run in place for 1 minute. After exercising, drink an 11-ounce glass of chilled mineral water with a thin lemon slice.

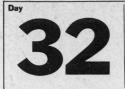
Thursday

Evening

Dinner menu (491 calories)
*Shrimp Creole (241 calories)
½ cup cooked white rice (112 calories)
1 medium stalk broccoli, steamed (18 calories) and sprinkled with 1 teaspoon lemon juice (1 calorie)
Tossed green salad made from ¼ head iceberg lettuce, shredded (10 calories) and sprinkled with 1 tablespoon chopped parsley (2 calories); serve with 1 tablespoon low-calorie bleu-cheese dressing (12 calories)
½ cup unsweetened applesauce (55 calories), mixed with ½ teaspoon cinnamon and 1 tablespoon chopped walnuts (40 calories)
Coffee (regular or decaffeinated) or tea (no sugar or milk)

*Shrimp Creole

10 medium-sized shrimp (100 calories)
Salt
1 teaspoon margarine (33 calories)
3 scallions, thinly sliced (12 calories)
1 clove garlic, minced (3 calories)
1 stalk celery, chopped (5 calories)
½ green pepper, chopped (8 calories)

1 can (8 ounces) tomato sauce (80 calories)
¼ teaspoon basil
¼ teaspoon thyme
1 bay leaf
1 cup water

Boil shrimp in lightly salted water for 3 minutes or, if frozen, cook according to package directions. Put margarine in a flameproof casserole over medium-high heat. Add scallions, garlic, celery, and green pepper. Cook for 2 minutes, stirring constantly. Add tomato sauce, basil, thyme, and bay leaf and bring to a boil. Add water, bring to a boil again, lower heat to very low, and simmer for 25 minutes. Add shrimp and cook for 5 minutes more. Serve over rice.

Note: Prepare mint tea and chill in refrigerator overnight to use for afternoon break on Day 33.

Beauty break: **fashion checklist and plan.** Generally, women who look the best and who enjoy fashion the most have learned how to add a few terrific-looking clothes to their wardrobe every season. They think before they buy and plan so that they can coordinate new things with old. One does not have to be rich to achieve a certain style and flair within a reasonable budget. Awareness and planning are the keys. Women who are aware keep up with the best fashion magazines; they know what looks good on them (but they are not afraid to experiment), and they plan well. An example of sound planning is buying a coat in a classic style and color at a holiday coat sale or at the end of the season. Coat styles rarely change drastically from year to year, and it makes sense to get the best possible coat at the most reasonable price. You will lose 10 pounds by following this diet and therefore you will be one size smaller. Now is a good time to go through your wardrobe and see what works and what doesn't. Have the becoming things altered and give away those things you don't like and never wear. And plan to add one or two new things to show off your slim new figure.

You will need: pencil and notebook.

Make this notebook your clothes diary. Use it for periodic reviews, for planning each new season, and for deciding what to take on any vacation or business trips. After you have weeded out all the clothes you plan to give away, list those you are keeping in the notebook. Do this by categories: skirts, pants, tops, sweaters, dresses, evening clothes, coats, shoes, accessories. List only clothes you love, that look well on you, and that are in good condition. French women as well as other Europeans often have fewer clothes than the American woman and yet manage to look more fashionable. One of their secrets is that they buy better quality clothes. Also, they make sure that pants and skirts really fit. You can adopt this same system and then vary your look by layering and by wearing accessories imaginatively. You should always have one or two very good sweaters—perhaps black and beige or black and dark red. If you concentrate on building a small but smashing-looking wardrobe you will find you are happier with your clothes. And you can achieve this fashion-wise look without devoting great chunks of your time and your money to it.

Eleven o'clock exercise break: mat exercises to relax you and tone your muscles.

Straight leg stretch

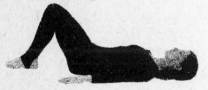

1. Lie on your back, arms at sides and knees bent with feet flat on floor.

2. Bring right knee to your chest.

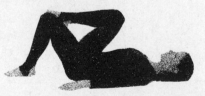

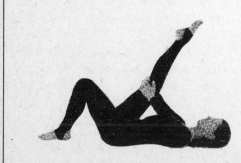

3. Straighten leg and grasp with hands. Pull leg toward you. Release and return to starting position.

4. Repeat with left leg. Alternate, lifting each leg 3 times.

Friday

Morning

On arising: **breathing exercise.** Stand by the side of the bed with feet together, spine erect, and shoulders relaxed. Begin the exercise by exhaling completely. You should be able to hear the exhalation. Next, inhale slowly and deeply through your nostrils. Your mouth should be closed. As you breathe in, lift your rib cage and contract your abdominal muscles. Fill lungs to capacity. Hold breath for a moment. Then exhale slowly and steadily until you feel you have completely emptied your lungs. Keep abdominal muscles contracted. Again, wait for a moment, and then inhale and repeat the exercise. Do this 10 times.

Immediately after breathing exercise: **wake-up exercises.**

Full extension twist

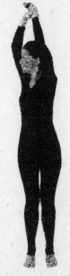

1. Stand with feet together, arms at sides. Breathing in, rise up on toes, lifting arms, linking fingers, and turning up palms.

2. Slowly twist body to right as far as is comfortable. Return to center, lower heels to floor.

3. Repeat, twisting to the left. Twist 5 times to each side.

Running in place. Always run on a carpeted or padded surface. Warm up by jogging very slowly for 50 steps. Rest for a moment and then run at a faster pace for 5 minutes. Lift feet 4 inches off the floor. Cool down by walking around, taking long strides, until your pulse rate and breathing have returned to normal.

Weigh yourself and record your weight. Congratulations!

Breakfast menu (232 calories)
1 4-ounce glass orange juice (55 calories)
1 egg, poached (78 calories)
½ hamburger bun, toasted (55 calories)
1 4-ounce glass skim milk (44 calories)
Coffee (regular or decaffeinated) or tea (no sugar)

Brown-bag lunch: If you are taking lunch to your office, prepare it right after breakfast.

Note: Transfer filet mignon from freezer to refrigerator.

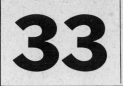

Friday

Daytime

Midmorning break: **herb tea.**

Lunch menu (318 calories)
*Open-faced chicken sandwich (273 calories)
½ cup canned apricots, water-packed (45 calories)
Coffee (regular or decaffeinated) or tea (no sugar or milk)

*Open-faced chicken sandwich

Baked chicken breast, sliced (prepared on Day 31) (147 calories)
2 leaves romaine lettuce (5 calories)
4 cucumber slices (5 calories)

1 tablespoon diet or imitation mayonnaise (48 calories)
1 slice whole wheat bread (68 calories)

Lightly toast the bread and spread on mayonnaise. Put lettuce leaves on bread, then cucumbers and chicken.

Midafternoon break: Run in place for 1 minute. Relax afterwards with a glass of cold mint tea with a thin slice of orange.

Friday

Evening

Dinner menu (512 calories)

1 11-ounce glass mineral water with ice and a thin slice of lemon
*Broiled steak with mushrooms (341 calories)
2 carrots, sliced and boiled (34 calories) and sprinkled with 2 teaspoons
  lemon juice (2 calories) and 1 teaspoon chopped parsley
½ cup green beans, steamed (21 calories) and sprinkled with 1 sliced scallion
  (4 calories)
Tossed green salad made from 2 cups Boston and romaine lettuce leaves,
  torn into bite-sized pieces (15 calories) and 4 sliced radishes (7 calories);
  serve with 1 tablespoon low-calorie bleu-cheese dressing (12 calories)
1 orange, peeled and sliced into 2 tablespoons orange juice and sprinkled
  with cinnamon (76 calories)
Coffee (regular or decaffeinated) or tea (no sugar or milk)

*Broiled steak and mushrooms

1 4-ounce filet mignon (275 calories) ⅓ cup beef broth, made from beef
5 mushrooms (25 calories)   bouillon cube (2 calories)
1 scallion, thinly sliced (4 calories)   1 tablespoon parsley, chopped
1 teaspoon margarine (33 calories)   (2 calories)
1 teaspoon Worcestershire sauce

Remove all fat from steak. Broil 4 inches from flame, about 5 minutes on each side.
While you are broiling steak, make mushroom sauce. Melt margarine in a nonstick
frying pan over high heat. Add sliced mushrooms and scallion. Cook for 2 minutes,
turning mushrooms to cook evenly. Pour Worcestershire sauce and beef broth over
mushrooms. Cook for 2 minutes. When steak is done, put on serving plate, pour
mushrooms over it and sprinkle with parsley.

Eleven o'clock exercise break: mat exercises to relax you and tone your
muscles.

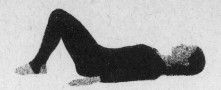

Straight leg stretch

1. Lie on your back, arms at sides and knees bent with feet flat on floor.

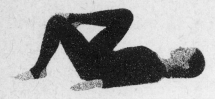

2. Bring right knee to your chest.

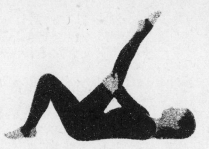

3. Straighten leg and grasp with hands. Pull leg toward you. Release and return to starting position.

4. Repeat with left leg. Alternate, lifting each leg 3 times.

Last thing before you go to bed: **relaxation technique.** Read through the exercise before you start.

Lie flat on your back on the mat. Legs should be relaxed. Arms are close to your sides, palms of hands facing up. Close your eyes and take two deep breaths. With your mind's eye, you are going to touch each part of your body and relax it. Start with your toes. Imagine you can touch your big toe with your mind; relax it. Move from toe to toe on the right foot. Then, as though your mind had a kind of relaxing ray, move up to the right ankle, the shin, the knee, the thigh. Now do your left foot and leg. Slowly cover the entire body, including the top of the head, the ears, the back of the head, the nape of the neck, and the spine, always focusing the beam of your mind on each part of your body to relax it. When you have finished, lie quietly for a few minutes and concentrate on your deep breathing.

Congratulations! You've done it! Make this weekend a time of celebration. Buy yourself something smashing to wear that will show off your slim new figure. Sign up for a dance class to learn to enjoy your body even more. Treat yourself well. That means you should continue your healthy, well-balanced new way of eating. Plan your weekend with this in mind, but allow yourself to increase your calorie intake a bit (add another slice of bread at breakfast or lunch, treat yourself to a midafternoon fruit or fruit juice break, have a slice of angelfood cake (just one slice). In general, stay away from sweets and fats as much as possible. If you do this, you will be able to maintain your new weight without a struggle. Enjoy the good life!